JINXED!

LAUGHING IN THE FACE OF
ALZHEIMER'S

MARLENE JAXON

Jinxed!
Laughing in the Face of Alzheimer's
By: Marlene Jaxon
www. MarleneJaxon.com

Copyright © 2019 by Honu Publishing
First Edition 2019

Editing by Caitlin Jackson
Book design by Project Whimsy, LLC.
Cover design by Stacy Coleman

ISBN: 9781706496359

My deepest love and gratitude
To Harold and Caitlin —
Together, they are the sole reason
this book exists

CONTENTS

A NOTE TO THE READER

My pushy daughter made me write this book. Let me rephrase that, since nobody makes *me* do anything. My very persuasive daughter, Caitlin, *urged* me to write this book. "You had a creative, upbeat way of caring for grandma. And the relationship the two of you had was certainly unique too. You should share your ideas with other people, Mom." I couldn't argue with her. Kids today!

It was never my choice to become knowledgeable about Alzheimer's. Alzheimer's chose me. So, like many people, I had to make the best of it. In the six years I spent as caregiver to my mother, Jinx, humor was indisputably the greatest *inner* resource I had. Always free and readily available, it required no doctor's referral or insurance approval. Believe me, it's not easy to find the 'lighter side" of dementia symptoms, but sometimes that's all you can do to maintain your sanity. Laughter became my most powerful survival tool in overcoming the difficult challenges we faced together each day.

Viewing mom's illness through the lens of humor not only sparked my creativity, but also my spontaneity, which was necessary for living in the present moment with mom. People with dementia live in the "now," just like children do. When I allowed myself to do the same, something wonderful happened – I felt like a kid again too. Daily playfulness ensued. Even though my mother passed away five years ago, I continue to enjoy living in the fully present state of mind I learned through her. Thanks, Ma!

While engaged in the most difficult undertaking of my life, another lovely unexpected benefit developed, in the form of a more enlightened mother-daughter relationship. As she and I gradually reversed roles – under the most adverse conditions – I could finally reconcile my past grievances by viewing my mother through new eyes.

I hope the story of how my family joined together in Jinx's final years proves helpful and uplifting to those "chosen" to be the caregiver of a dementia patient. Although everybody's experience will be different, there are plenty of commonalities: Seemingly insurmountable challenges and sacrifice, insanely difficult daily decisions, unparalleled frustration, unending medical appointments, and the heart-wrenching, insidious loss of the individual we love. But, remember, we also share the indominable human spirit, and there are some amazing silver linings to be found if we look for them.

INTRODUCTION
My New "Normal"

Is mom still alive in there?

Her bedroom door remains closed at 9 am. My tall, kitchen barstool provides me with an unobstructed view of it. I sip a second cup of coffee from my perch, staring intently at her doorknob – willing it to move with my thoughts. *Turn, damn it!* Mom has been in her room for twelve hours now, but that's no longer unusual; she doesn't always come out on her own anymore, even after she's awake. Sometimes she remains in bed, always on her back now, smiling up at the ceiling in wonderment – like a child searching for shapes in the clouds.

My 86-year-old mother, Jinx Scribner, has Alzheimer's, congestive heart failure, and severe sleep apnea. Each morning brings with it, upon opening her bedroom door, the very real possibility of discovering she has passed away during the night. As morbid as it sounds, I already have a pretty good idea what her lifeless form would look like. Quite regularly, mom nods off on the couch in front of the TV – her head tilted back, mouth agape, hands neatly folded across her belly, and eerily still. Whenever that happens, I instinctively put a palm to her chest, feeling for her heartbeat and the shallow rise and fall of her breathing. This little ritual – one I had initially thought of as macabre – has now become routine.

Staring down at my two canine kids, snoozing soundly at my feet, I sigh and set my mug of now-cold coffee on the counter. "What do you say, guys? Shall we go check on your grandma?"

No reply, as usual.

My neck and shoulders tighten as I approach mom's room. Same thing, different day; tormented by the same two agonizing questions: *Is she still alive in there? Do I want her to be?* Both possibilities make me cringe because hoping for either one carries an unbearable level of guilt.

Wouldn't it be better if mom simply passed away peacefully in her sleep? The argument seems selfless on the surface. I want to spare her the final grim phase of the cruel brain disease, when she will basically be reduced to an infant; no longer able to walk, talk, chew, or even swallow. I'd say mom's present cognitive age is approximately that of a two-year-old. The current demands her care places upon the three of us – her daughter, her son-in-law, and her granddaughter would mortify the proud mother I used to know. Undeniably, given the choice and with sound mind, she would *rather* die.

Admittedly, hoping for a sudden, peaceful demise during the night isn't solely about ending *her* misery. There is no denying that, I too, want to be spared the pain of witnessing the horror of mom's end-stage Alzheimer's. My fear of it runs deep. I also yearn to have my old, carefree life back – one which doesn't involve caring for a 140lb. toddler, 24/7. At age 53, I am easily two decades past the required level of maternal energy and enthusiasm. At five years and counting, the daily uncertainty of when the four of us will finally be freed from our current reality is maddening. Even a prison sentence comes with an approximate release date.

I have only one counterargument against discovering my mother has passed away in her sleep, and it is equally self-centered: I'm not quite ready to let her go yet. Hell, I can't even bring myself to send her to a nursing home. Mom's dementia has gifted her with a lovely, childlike demeanor. She isn't combative, belligerent, suspicious, or angry. She is a sweet, little girl – *my* little girl. And although our roles are now oddly reversed, she will still always be my *mother* too. I'm not ready to part with her. I doubt I ever will be.

So, on this particular day, like most days, I hope to find mom either snoring her head off or wide awake – staring at a heavenly sight only she can see. Wiping the sweat from my hand before timidly turning the knob, I crack the door open just enough to peek into my mother's bedroom – the room in our home, built specifically for her, twenty years ago.

She's still alive. Thank God!

Relief floods my being and relaxes my muscles. Unaware of my presence, mom is sitting on the edge of the bed, partially wrapped in her chenille bedspread, staring blankly down at her feet. There's no telling how long she's been there like that – two minutes or two hours. I walk over to her and gently comb the wispy strands of gray hair away from her face with my fingers.

"Good morning Princess Jinx! Did you sleep well m' lady?" I lean over and kiss her on the forehead.

She looks up and smiles at me. I love that sweet smile.

"Yeah," she nods.

"Were you dreaming about your handsome fella, Bill, again last night?" I give her a sly wink.

A spark of mischief flickers in her eyes at the mere mention of Bill's name, followed by a sly grin.

"Oh yeah," she beams and giggles with the embarrassment of a teenage girl.

Bill, my father, had been her husband for thirty-five years and the one and only love of her life. But her memory of him now is as her boyfriend, with zero knowledge of wedding him or bearing his four children. Blissfully unaware he died in 1982, she never asks his whereabouts.

I bow before her, in an exaggerated, courtly curtsy, and extend my hand to assist her in rising from the bed.

"May I escort you to the royal potty, your Highness?" I ask, in my most haughty British accent.

"Okay, Joanie," she agrees, as she slips her hand in mine.

There's no point in telling her Joanie is a cousin who lives in Idaho...or that my name is Marlene. As long as she knows I love her, I don't care what she calls me.

I pull my mother to a standing position and walk her into the adjacent bathroom. Her cotton pajamas sag with the weight of her saturated, nighttime diaper. I've become quite adept at expediting mom's morning toileting routine. Ten minutes is all I need to get her clean and dry enough for breakfast. Three cheers for adult pull-ups!

Mom grips my forearm for balance as we head to the kitchen; she's forgotten how to use her cane. I slide a chair out for her and make sure she's comfortably seated. As I do, I notice the bowl containing decorative fruit in the middle of the table is amiss; a bright yellow, paper mâché peach has a sizable bite taken out of it. Evidently, it was ravaged in the wee hours by somebody in their quest for a midnight snack. The alleged culprit is sitting right under my nose, so I playfully interrogate her – with obvious lightheartedness – so she knows I'm not angry.

"Did you eat this peach last night, Ma?"

Mom's face lights up with a proud smile, "Yup!"

"Well," I prompt her, "how did it taste?"

She thinks about it for a few seconds before snickering, "Not too bad."

"So, what would you like for your breakfast today?"

"Peaches!" she declares with glee.

"Paper or plastic, Ma'am?" This joke is strictly for me. My mother no longer comprehends sarcasm and stares at me unphased. I throw open the fridge door and survey its contents.

"Wouldn't you rather have eggs?" I bring them over to her and flip the lid on the carton. Showing her the eggs helps her understand what I'm talking about.

"Okay." She reaches for one to eat.

"How 'bout I cook them first, Ma?"

"Oh yeah," she snickers again.

Her laughter ignites my own. At this late stage in her disease, I know she probably has no memory of chewing a hole in the fake fruit during the night, but it's still fun to engage her in a conversation about it. I also realize paper mâché munchies can no longer be left out on the kitchen table, so I make a mental note to hide them a little later.

As diligent as I try to be, I can't anticipate *every* safeguard necessary to protect my mother, but I don't waste any mental energy chastising myself for it anymore. It's not possible to fully childproof a house from the antics of an adult-size youngster. Could mom have choked while grazing on the paper mâché peach? Yes. But she didn't. There's no sense beating myself up about it. Some of the balls I'm juggling are going to hit the floor. I'm doing the best I can. I've also learned to see the humor in the absurd. I smile to myself as I recall an amusing, little-known tidbit: Papier mâché is French for chewed paper.

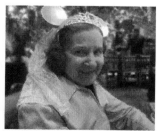

Princess Jinx's Disneyland birthday celebration – Thanksgiving 2011

MOM'S ROOM

A few weeks after mom's passing, I once again found myself hesitantly facing her bedroom, this time with a different, but still painful, challenge. I needed to begin the daunting task of sorting through all her belongings and deciding what to do with each and every item: *Who gets what? What goes to charity? What do I do with all those knickknacks?*

I was lucky, actually. Some people have an entire house full of stuff to assess and pack. It was then that a poignant realization came over me. The contents of my mother's entire life – 87 years on this earth – had been reduced to occupying one small room of our Arizona home. Sure, there were a few pieces scattered throughout our house: Her old steamer trunk made a funky end table in the family room and her cast iron frying pans were still cooking up tasty pancakes. Even her own mother's garnet-colored, etched-glass vase beautified our dining room – with or without flowers in it. However, most of Jinx's possessions were contained within the four walls of her 12-by-12 bedroom.

I knew sifting through mom's things would be a slow and emotional process for me, but I chose to do it alone. If any of my three siblings – Karen, Billy, or Jaime – had asked to join me, I'm sure I would have let them. Perhaps they had been politely awaiting my invitation and I forgot to extend one. I admit to selfishly not giving them any real consideration, seeking instead, to satisfy the overpowering need to savor every remaining piece of my mother's life, on my own terms. I wanted quiet, private time to be alone with her; with the many special memories I kept inside the little room – Mom's room. I just needed to summon up the courage.

I entered tentatively, as I had done hundreds of times the past couple of years. Maybe it was a habit now. Standing in the doorway, I struggled to survey the surroundings through suddenly moist eyes and a twisting ache in my gut. Of course, I'd gone inside numerous times since she'd passed away the month before, but I'd purposely always made it quick – only darting in to retrieve a necessary legal or financial document. Never allowing myself to *feel* the room; to feel her presence. I flat-out avoided her. But now, I decided, it was time to face the obligatory music. Mom and I needed to "take a meeting," as they say in the business world. It was time to reconcile my heart with reality. *I would absolutely, positively NEVER see her in THIS bedroom EVER again.*

My dread soon turned to smiles once the obvious set in – the room was a joyful reflection of her, and I could indeed feel her in every square inch of the space. My mother's possessions revealed so much about who she was. A cursory glance around the room was all it took to recognize exactly what mattered most to her in her life. I took a deep breath, stretched out across mom's bed, and basked in the midst of everything she had held dear.

Nothing conveyed the modest, sentimental tastes of my mother more than her bedroom furniture – the same faux-walnut set she and my dad bought when they moved from New Jersey to Arizona in 1973. Although over 40 years-old and constructed from cheap, flimsy particle board, to her it was irreplaceable; *they* picked it out together as they began their exciting, new adventure in the Grand Canyon State. The cozy, full-size bed was the one she shared with Bill. She would *never* think of owning a different one. Sleeping in *that* bed, was tantamount to sleeping with *him*. I closed my eyes and pictured the two of them lying there asleep in each other's arms.

The matching dresser and nightstand were adorned with mom's charming collection of angel and hummingbird knickknacks, neatly arranged on embroidered doilies. An array of whimsical jewelry boxes, of various shapes and sizes, sat clustered atop her chest of drawers. The ornate, maple wood box, displayed in the very center, instantly caught my eye. I pensively caressed the intricately carved design in the lid, knowing *that* particular one played my parent's favorite love song – *Somewhere, My Love*. I wasn't sure my heart could bear listening to it, but before I could change my mind, I gave the key on the bottom a couple of quick turns and lifted the top.

The tinkling, romantic melody swirled out of the red velvet interior as I examined mom's precious "valuables" within. The miniature treasure chest brimmed with an assortment of tangled chains, daddy's old tie clips, cuff links, and tarnished watchbands. There was nothing flashy or materialistic about mom. Her "priceless" jewelry consisted mainly of heart and rainbow pendants – the kind a proud grandma wears around her neck. And she did indeed wear them – even the plastic ones. Since the loss of her husband, all rainbows had come to symbolize him saying, "Hi Hon!" from heaven. Tears welled up in my eyes again, as the tender, little tune flowed into my memories. Damn that love song! It got me every time. I closed the lid, set the box aside, and released the inevitable floodwaters into a fistful of tissues. My mother always kept Kleenex in her room. "Thanks, Ma," I sniffled. Closing my eyes again, I imagined her arms around me and took a few minutes to remember how comforting her hugs always were.

Once composed, I went over to the single window in the bedroom and slid aside the pink, homemade curtains to let in some natural light. A talented seamstress, mom had put many miles on the old Singer sewing machine, whose cabinet now served as a TV stand. Pausing to admire my

8

mother's handiwork up close, I realized she had flawlessly handstitched the curtains. *Jeesh! Where did she get the patience, not to mention the keen eyesight?*

Of course, Jinx didn't *need* to sew her own curtains, by hand or otherwise; she simply couldn't see the sense in buying something she could easily make herself. She had always been sensible, thrifty, and resourceful – worthy traits which had *not* rubbed off on me. Ditto for her sewing prowess. It usually took me an hour to hem one pant leg of my jeans, only to have it come undone after the third washing.

I loved how my mother used corresponding window treatments and bedding to alternately dress her bedroom for winter and summer. In the summer she hung the breezy, sky blue curtains (also handstitched!) and covered her bed with a fluffy blue, chenille bedspread. In the winter, she replaced the blue drapes with the warmer-toned, pink ones and switched the bedcover to a rosy, ruffled comforter. Regardless of the season, she always kept the same tidy arrangement of decorative throw pillows on the bed because each had been a gift from a beloved child.

Speaking of children, Jinx's bedroom was practically a shrine to all the cherished cherubs in her life. She proudly displayed dozens of pictures of her kids, grandkids, and great grandkids everywhere she possibly could. They hung from every wall and sat on every dresser. She even devoted the entire entryway to her room, resembling a mini gallery, to photos of all the youngsters she had babysat over the years. She called them "her kids" and loved them as her own. In turn, they referred to her as "their other mother." Three exceptional girls, whom Jinx helped raise from infants to teens, attended mom's 80th birthday party, and stayed in close contact with her right up to the end. You can't help but admire and respect such a deep, lifelong bond.

Despite not being devoutly Catholic, mom's bedroom showcased her reverence for Jesus Christ and the Virgin Mary. Statues, portraits, crucifixes, and rosary beads figured prominently in the décor – resembling a Christian gift store. Personally, I wouldn't have been able to sleep with all those holy eyeballs peering down on me in the darkness, but mom slept peacefully in the belief of their divine protection.

Judging by the myriad of religious icons on display – practically wall-to-wall angels – one would never guess Jinx hadn't been to Catholic mass in over twenty years. On occasion, mom was even known to "take thy Lord's name in vain" with exclamations of, "For Chrissakes!" and "Goddammit!" I didn't see the contradiction as hypocritical. Mom never preached, proselytized or claimed to be perfect. Jinx Scribner was a *good* woman – definitely heaven material in my book. If *she* couldn't get in, nobody could!

Standing at my mother's headboard, I smiled up at the obvious focal point of her room: The colorful, lifelike painting of Jinx and Bill, hanging squarely on the wall above her bed for two decades. My artistic husband, Harold, had rendered the poster-size artwork from one of mom's all-time favorite photos taken at their surprise 25th wedding anniversary party in 1972. The moment captured on canvas is of the happy couple's joyful embrace, right after daddy slipped a new wedding band on his delighted wife's finger. He's pulling her close against his chest, their hands entwined together. They're both laughing – my father so hard his eyes are shut. It's a perfect snapshot of an idyllic slice of time. One I'll never forget, though I was only twelve. Reflecting back on it, I don't remember anything else about the celebration; only that moment. The vivid painting has kept it alive for me, all these years.

Harold created the portrait for Jinx shortly after she lost her dear husband of thirty-five years. Naturally, she cherished it, as do I, which is why it still hangs prominently where it always has: On the same wall, directly above the bed (albeit a new one), in the same 12-by-12 space in our

10

home, which no matter how we decorate it or furnish it, will forever be known as "Mom's room."

Time flew by while reminiscing with mom that afternoon. My fear had been all for naught. And despite the sentimental distractions, I actually made respectable headway with regards to sorting her belongings. At the end of the day, as I shut my mother's bedroom door, an old familiar theme song came to mind, one sung by a favorite performer of mine and mom's – Miss Carol Burnett:

I'm so glad we had this time together,
just to have a laugh or sing a song.
Seems we just get started and before you know it,
comes the time we have to say…so long.

Goodnight, Ma. (earlobe tug)

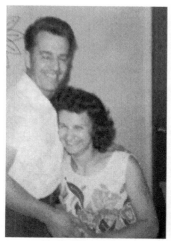 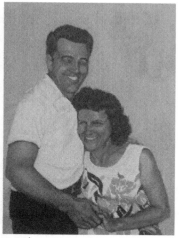

Left: *Original photo taken at their 25ᵗʰ wedding anniversary party*
Right: *Portrait Harold painted that still hangs in "Mom's Room"*

THE SCRIBNER CLAN

I have to laugh when I hear some people's reaction to my mother's nickname of Jinx.

"Jinx? What a cool name! She sounds like a such fun mom."

They automatically presume she was a spirited person of mischief, spontaneity, and adventure. They picture a sexy spitfire in a low-cut polka dot dress, dashing from one party to the next; the center of attention, a coquettish flirt captivating all the men in attendance. My laugher comes from the humorous fact that mom was *nothing* like that – not in *any* way. I might even venture to say Jinx may possibly have been one of the most cautious, conservative, rigid, and boring (sorry Ma!) people I knew.

My mother's biggest vice was *not* having any vices. She never indulged in anything. Even during the "swinging '60s" she never drank an alcoholic drink or smoked. Which, to her credit, is probably why she lived so long! Mom always had flimsy excuses for not having fun, but as an idealistic kid, I gave it my best shot every year when I badgered her with the same three requests.

"Can I *please* join the Girl Scouts, Mom? My friends are learning a lot of cool things."

"Not on your life!" She'd wrinkle up her nose in disgust. "You don't want to do that – you'll have to clean fish."

"Can I *please* have my friends over for a birthday party, Mommy? They always invite me to theirs, and they get so many more presents."

"Yeah right!" She'd scoff. "You think I want a bunch of kids over? Get outta here!"

"Can daddy and I *please* bake Christmas cookies from scratch and decorate them? We promise we'll clean up!"

"You're not messing up my kitchen!" Then she'd pull out a log of packaged Pillsbury "slice-off" cookie dough from the fridge and slam it down on the countertop. "Here you go. These are just as good."

Does that *sound* like a spirited, spontaneous individual? Mom's given name of "Josephine" always seemed more fitting to me. It conjured up the image of an old-fashioned girl; someone sensible, reliable, practical, and frugal – a much more accurate description of my mother. Her family called her "Josie" for short.

Josie didn't acquire the nickname "Jinx" until high school, when a school chum flippantly gave it to her. In class one day, the young man jokingly announced to their fellow classmates, "Josie is a jinx! I have bad luck whenever she's around!" The rest is history. With one silly, off-the-cuff proclamation, from that day forward, and for the remainder of her life, Josephine would be known as "Jinx." The fellow's words also led to mom's sincere belief that the number thirteen – associated with the bad luck superstition – brought her good fortune. She considered Friday the 13th her lucky day!

Jinx's greatest source of pride came from caring for her husband, children, and home. I believe if I surveyed my three siblings, we'd all agree we preferred having a sensible mother we could depend upon, rather than a party flirt. She was *always* there for us: Every day when we awoke, got off the school bus, ate dinner, had nightmares, got sick, and through all of life's problems.

13

I never heard anybody call my father, Vincent William Scribner, anything other than "Bill." His mother even referred to him as Bill throughout her will, which resulted in him having to prove his identity. Daddy was a 5'6", stocky, little wisecracking prankster who loved joking around and playing tricks on people. He had a perpetual spark of mischief in his baby-blue eyes and an infectious zest for life. He used to practice rock-n-roll and blues riffs on his electric, Fender Stratocaster guitar downstairs in the playroom. With his white undershirt, thick dark pompadour, and Camel cigarette dangling from his lips, he had a bit of a rebel bad-boy thing going on. He enjoyed juicy steaks, pork chops, Jersey corn and tomatoes, and *every* kind of dessert. Booze was limited to the Christmas season only – when he would indulge in ONE whiskey highball.

My dad had a generosity of spirit which enabled us to see exactly who he was – and adore him, warts and all. But sometimes, I saw a bit *too* much when he'd parade around the house in his stretched-out "tighty whities" (more like loosie goosies), leaving little to the imagination. My father wore his emotions on his sleeve at all times; he could weep openly, hug freely, roll on the floor with laughter, and punch a door in anger. He hid nothing. Bill was the opposite of Jinx in many ways; unfortunately, that also included his lifespan.

Despite my dad being the breadwinner of the family (usually the person with the power), my mom was the helmsman of our lives – in charge of everything – displaying unwavering strength and competence. When I wanted someone to play with, or make me laugh, nobody was more fun than daddy. When I needed comfort or help with a serious matter, I ran to mom. He was the silly, spontaneous parent, and she was the unyielding, reliable rock. They were the perfect balance for one another.

While growing up, the relationship I had with my siblings was not one of particular closeness, mostly due to our ages and the varied way we were each raised.

My sister, Karen, born in 1948, had a simpler, more innocent upbringing. The twelve-year age difference between us made me view her more like an aunt or an extra adult in the house. Karen graduated high school in 1966 – the year I finished kindergarten. I don't remember ever playing with her, or even interacting with her much; she was either working or out with friends, like most teenagers.

We shared a spacious attic bedroom, but I had explicit directions not to touch *anything* of hers. I pretended to despise her Beatles posters, while harboring a secret crush on Paul McCartney. I'm sure she was thrilled about having a child's full-size playhouse in her room.

Karen got married and moved out, at age twenty-three, when I was only eleven. I remember being so relieved and thankful to her boyfriend, Ken, for proposing to her. Twenty-three seemed positively ancient to me, prompting my genuine fear she would remain an "old maid" forever. Upon hearing the exciting news of her engagement, I immediately ran to each of my friends' homes to tell them, like a town crier: "Hear ye, hear ye! Karen Scribner saved from eternal spinsterhood!" We still joke about this at our family gatherings.

My older brother, Billy, had a completely different upbringing. As the firstborn son, he was hailed by my dad's side of the family as the second coming of Christ in 1954. They celebrated "Little Bill," with undue praise, money, and adoration, for the certain distinction of carrying on the Scribner family name. Nobody could anticipate the real possibility of him siring only daughters – which he ultimately did.

Six years separated us, so he wasn't much of a playmate either. He mostly skulked around my friends and me, teasing and tormenting us to the point of tears. Billy seemed, in my mind, to be the central focus of my parents' daily lives. They were always engaged in a serious problem regarding either his failing grades and/or his incorrigible behavior.

To remedy the situation, evidently the only course of action they could come up with, was for mom to regularly beat him with a leather strap and daddy to reward him with even *more* money plus expensive gifts (i.e. a drum set and mini-bike). For some curious reason, this INSANE method of discipline failed to correct their son's behavior. As a final desperate measure, they allowed him to drop out of high school *and* vocational school. Even back then, I was not too young to see how ludicrous and dysfunctional Billy's upbringing was.

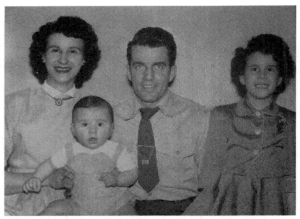

Mom, Billy, Daddy, & Karen – circa 1955

Only two years my junior, I finally found a buddy in my brother Jaime. We rarely got into trouble, not because we were perfect little angels, but because we were too damn terrified of our mother's leather strap to misbehave. However, with mom and daddy usually preoccupied with Billy's problems, my little bro and I could easily fly under the radar.

16

Most of my warmest childhood memories involve Jaime. We ice skated and sledded together, went trick-or-treating in homemade costumes, fished on the canal banks and biked around the neighborhood, enjoying summer fairs. We each had our own friends, but we were still constant companions.

Unlike Billy, Jaime was never celebrated for the possibility of carrying on the Scribner family name, which he was the only one of us to do. I don't think the slight bothered Jaime much. His easy-going nature made him a low-maintenance kid and a happy-go-lucky adult.

From a young age, my parents labeled me "the smart one." I was their child who walked at eight months of age, spoke in full sentences before two, earned straight-A's in school, and graduated college. They held high expectations of me, and I always delivered.

Speaking of delivery, my breech birth was the most difficult and the most expensive (a whopping $200!) for my parents, requiring four doctors to bring me into the world. It was so dangerous, when introducing me to strangers, mom would refer to me as *the kid who almost killed her*. I have to confess to loving the story and the title; the moniker of "troublemaker" suits me fine, as does my grand entrance in 1960.

According to legend, I had traveled too far down the birth canal for a C-section to be safely performed. To make matters worse, I was sliding into home plate butt-first, with both a leg and an arm outstretched. My mother was "knocked-out," (as she put it) and knew nothing of the peril. My poor father was asked which life he wanted saved in the possible event of losing mother or child. The decision had to be a painful one for him to make, but I doubt he thought twice about it. Bill chose Jinx, the woman he adored, and the mother of his two other children. I've never held it against my dad because I believe he made the correct decision.

Mom unashamedly admitted she decided to have me to "give her something to do." With her other kids in school full-time, the obvious answer for filling the long, tedious days was taking caring of another baby – yours truly. It's nice to know I was planned…similar to a rainy-day activity. I'm not complaining – I'm thrilled mom saw no other options!

WHAT'S THE MATTER WITH MOM?

I'm often asked by fellow caregivers, "When was the first time you noticed something *not quite right* going on with your mother? On that matter, my family is 100% in agreement. It had to be the rainy evening, in January of 2008, when mom returned home from a Sunday outing with my sister, Karen. We believe that fateful day to be the onset of her gradual mental decline and the prelude to our unique journey together.

Karen usually brought mom home before dark. The winter sun setting an hour earlier, plus the wet weather, gave me slight cause for worry. Upon hearing the front door open, I ran to the entryway to greet them, only to be knocked speechless by my mother's ghastly appearance as she shuffled slowly into the house, gripping Karen's elbow for support. She looked like she'd been in a barroom brawl: Her cheek bruised, and her arm in a sling, her facial affect totally blank with her mouth hanging slack-jawed.

"Oh my God! What happened? Are you okay, Ma?"

She didn't acknowledge me in any way.

"Mom slipped and fell in the mall parking lot," Karen's voice cracked with fatigue. "I took her to the ER, and the doctor said she dislocated her shoulder. They gave her oxygen and some pain meds."

"I guess I'm dopey," my mother finally spoke. She seemed dopey alright. I chalked it up to the pain pills and decided to direct all my questions to my sister.

"Did mom fall on her face? Did they x-ray her head ? Does she have a concussion or anything?" I had so many questions, but Karen didn't have many answers. She'd clearly had a rough day too.

"They did some kind of scan, but I guess everything's okay."

After my sister left, I combed through the ER paperwork and saw no mention of a concussion or brain injury of any kind. It still worried me, though, because I knew from my mother's bruised face she must have jolted her head to some degree.

A couple of weeks later, with no narcotics to blame, mom still sported a dazed and confused demeanor. I started wondering about the cause of her fall. *Maybe she didn't actually slip and fall? Maybe she had a small stroke and fell?* I scheduled an MRI for her, but it revealed nothing out of the ordinary. However, my mother was never *quite* the same again.

In the months following her fall, the most notable difference in Jinx was her refusal to do the home physical therapy exercises for her shoulder injury. It was strangely uncharacteristic of her to have no interest in regaining the full use of her arm and hand again. Only six months earlier (at age 80), after her hip replacement, mom had been so diligent and dedicated to her rehabilitation, that within 30 days of her surgery, she was scaling our staircase with the sure-footedness of a mountain goat.

The task of delivering mom to her PT appointments twice a week fell mainly to Karen and Billy, since neither of them worked, and their schedules were more flexible. At the time, I taught middle school science, and my brother Jaime worked in construction. Jinx cooperated fully with her therapists at the rehab facility, but no matter how much we all lectured her on the importance of also doing the home exercises, it never motivated her. We repeatedly and sternly stressed the necessity of stretching and strengthening her muscles and tendons. Our warnings about the possibility of her losing the range of motion in her arm did not faze her either. Mom remained steadfast and stubborn in her answer to us. She didn't want to do the exercises because it hurt. Plain and simple.

Every week, when Billy delivered her home from PT, he and I would sit her down and lecture her *again* on the probable consequences of not doing the home rehab work.

"You know your arm might freeze like that, Ma...all bent and crooked."

Each time she'd nod in agreement and promise to do her exercises – but she never actually would.

Like a naughty kid, mom began lying to us, adamantly insisting she did her exercises every day, while the three of us were gone. To confirm my suspicion about her inactivity, I purposely hung the resistance pulley and therapy bands in a specific arrangement on her closet door prior to leaving for work. When I checked it upon my return home – big surprise – I could see the exercise equipment had obviously not been touched.

Mom's lack of progress resulted in the denial of insurance coverage for further therapeutic treatments. By then, my patience had completely waned on the matter.

"I don't care if she *ever* goes to any more PT appointments. It's a waste of everyone's time and energy." I told Karen. I had had enough of trying to convince that stubborn old mule what was best for her. "If mom wants a crooked arm, so be it!"

My teaching job already consumed at least 60 hours of my week. By the time I fought the afternoon rush-hour traffic, I was pretty well-spent. Once home, the never-ending household chores demanded my attention. Adding 90 minutes of physical therapy exercises with mom to my list of obligations was out of the question. *Nope, not happening!*

I had to draw the line somewhere. Time with my teenage daughter and hard-working husband came first. And how about a little time for my own self-care? There were only so many hours in the day, and I'd never had any appreciation or patience for self-sacrificing martyrs.

What was with her anyway? My mother had always displayed an incredibly high tolerance for pain. When mom broke her hip the previous summer, she didn't even cry. Now that same woman was acting like a big weenie, claiming her arm exercises hurt? The incongruity baffled me, but I skeptically shrugged it off. *She's just becoming an obstinate old fart!*

Over the next year or so, despite a mountain of clues and evidence, I refused to recognize my mother's cognitive problems as anything other than old age. It's easy to fool yourself, since early signs of dementia can look a lot like "senior moments." I cringe at how much I rationalized the many changes in her behavior. Submerged in denial, I made excuse after excuse for her, until I finally couldn't.

Reflecting back on that time, when unmistakable changes in Jinx were occurring quite rapidly, I can't help but feel remiss for not recognizing a major problem much sooner than I did. However, I don't believe 100% of the blame belongs to me, since mom's own longtime physician never saw cause for concern or recommended any testing. Every time I mentioned my mother's apparent declining mental state during a visit, she poo-pooed my inquiries with, "Your mother is getting up there in age."

If I had been armed with greater knowledge on the subject, I would have been a more confident and assertive advocate for mom, right from the git-go. To be fair, a decade ago, Alzheimer's was not the "in your face" subject it is today. There wasn't a barrage of news articles, books, and movies on the topic. Nowadays, everybody knows somebody who's a caregiver or an actual patient. A steady stream of information abounds almost everywhere you look. Back then – not so much.

Still, I regret my ignorance, and I wish I would have been more forceful with the doctor, who only continued to enable my denial. All the signs for dementia were there. I guess I didn't want to see them. How could I not noticed the obvious changes in my mother's daily habits? That *alone* should have been enough warning. If ever there was a creature of *habit*, it was Jinx Scribner. Any deviation in her routine or behavior should have alerted me like a flaming flare-gun signal.

Every morning, mom got up no later than 7 o'clock. She ate her toast and drank her instant coffee while standing at the kitchen counter window, watching the birds in the backyard. Then she got dressed in the same polyester, stretch slacks and colorful blouse she'd worn since my earliest memories of her (circa 1963!).

After breakfast, mom made her bed and tidied her room. Then she'd sit in *her corner of the couch* (literally, nobody else was allowed to sit there), reading novels, doing puzzles, and the occasional needlework project. For lunch, she usually ate a bologna sandwich and drank a tiny glass of root beer, again while standing at the kitchen window. After school, she made a snack for Caitlin (yes, even through high school!). Then she helped prepare dinner, ate with us at the table, watched a little TV, and went to bed. That was her routine. Every. Single. Day.

Jinx also kept the same hairstyle for 70 years, from adolescence into her eighties. Never visiting a hair salon, she cut her own dark brown locks, always to the collar bone, and permed it herself. On Friday morning she washed it, set it in bobby pins, and wrapped it in a kerchief. The following morning she dismantled the works and brushed out the bouncy waves, which would last exactly one week.

Considering her predictability and consistency, I'm sure you're wondering what took me so long to notice my mother's obvious mental deterioration. Well, I *noticed* it. I just didn't *accept* it.

After mom's fall, her highly unusual lack of cleanliness caught my attention. Almost overnight, I had to remind her to bathe, wash her hair, brush her teeth, do laundry, and put on clean clothes. It should have been a humongous red flag. Instead, I brushed it off as probably an "old person thing." *A lot of old folks get a bit lackadaisical in their senior years.* But it did make me wonder further. *What else isn't she cleaning?*

A prompt inspection of mom's living area confirmed my suspicion of neglect: The sink and vanity in her bathroom were coated in hair and a layer of sticky, VO5 hairspray. The furnishings and knickknacks in her bedroom were solidly covered in dust. Mom had always prided herself on her housekeeping, so I knew something had to be wrong. One day, I finally asked her why she didn't clean anymore.

Mom looked up from her book and mulled it over for a second. Finally she shrugged, "I guess I don't think about it." Then she went back to reading.

Mentally, I continued to rationalize her behavior. *Maybe she's tired of doing housework. Surely an 81-year-old woman has earned the right to relax?*

Soon after, we noticed Jinx losing interest in her leisure activities, as well. All she seemed to do was watch TV. No more embroidery, gardening, or writing letters to friends. When Harold realized mom had stopped watering the flowers she had planted in the yard, he generously offered to build her a large, raised planter on our covered patio. He figured gardening in the shade, without having to bend over, might be more appealing to her. Oddly enough, she told him not to bother.

Maybe mom's feeling her age more than she's letting on.

In all our years together, I never knew how she *truly* felt. My mother never complained to anyone about anything. She preferred not to bother people with her troubles, so she pretended not to have any. Mom always

24

claimed to be either "good" or "fine," and everything around her was also always "good" or "fine." The older I got, the more her insipid answers annoyed me. Just once I wanted her to trust me by frankly admitting, "I'm tired today," or "I feel lousy" – something resembling genuine feelings instead of the brave face she wore to hide her actual needs. Now that mom was clearly experiencing cognitive difficulties, I felt even less in the mood for guessing games but held little hope of her sharing honest emotions with me when it wasn't something she ever did. The chances of her asking for help were slim to none.

In the following months, mom gradually lost her ability to prepare and cook dinner. I remember the final time she made her signature dish – stuffed cabbage – for us. A family favorite she probably prepared at least a hundred times since she was a girl, the simple Polish recipe was comprised of only three main ingredients; seasoned hamburger mixed with rice, wrapped in cabbage leaves. That evening at the dinner table, as soon as we each cut into our cabbage rolls, we started cracking up, including the cook herself.

"Uh...Ma,...where's the rice?"

"Uh-oh...did I forget to put it in?" Jinx seemed only mildly embarrassed.

Caitlin poked around the cabbage in her bowl with her fork. "Mine only has burger in the leaves, Grandma."

"You're getting kooky in your old age, Jinx," Harold chimed in.

Mom took a bite of her food and wrinkled her face in disgust.

"Not too good," she continued chewing. "Yep, I guess I'm losing my marbles," she chuckled. For the first time, I seriously contemplated that might actually be true.

It wasn't long before she couldn't figure out how to turn on the oven or stove, proclaiming, "All those knobs are too confusing." She refrained from cooking altogether, after that. Mom never expressed any frustration about her decline in skills – she merely stopped doing the things she usually did.

Although we severely missed Jinx's help at dinner time, I was glad she stopped cooking on her own rather than me having to put a halt to it for safety sake. Denying mom the pleasure of preparing meals for her family would have been tough for me to do, but I would have if necessary. I also counted my blessings she had quit driving way back in 1953, which meant I wouldn't have to deal with that touchy subject either. If she hadn't, I would have surely stripped her of car privileges around this time. Common sense dictates if a person doesn't have the mental fitness to remember a simple recipe or how to turn on a stove, then the question of operating a motor vehicle should be a nonnegotiable issue. Besides, how hard can it be to stop a person with memory issues from driving? In mom's case, all I would have had to do was hide her car keys, and she would have assumed she lost them.

As time went by, my mother's mental confusion also became evident in her attire: She started putting her bedroom slippers and sneakers on the wrong feet; forgetting to wear a bra (WAY out character for Mrs. Modesty!); and combining her slacks and blouses with pajama tops and bottoms. I wasn't bothered by the inappropriateness of her clothes – she wasn't leaving the house most days anyway – but it was disconcerting to see her once sharp mind short-circuiting.

I usually made light of her appearance by jokingly pointing out her odd wardrobe choices. "Nice outfit, Ma!" or "You might wanna harness those boobs, young lady!" Which always caused mom to look down at herself and laugh, "Oops! Oh boy, that's no good! I better change." Then, she'd head back to her bedroom to fix her fashion faux pas, and I would, once again, set my brain to "denial mode." *I guess that's probably normal for somebody her age...what's the harm in dressing silly anyway?*

26

Meanwhile, Harold and Caitlin started reporting their own worrisome observations to me. Caitlin came home from school a few times and found her grandma reading on the couch as usual – except with her book *upside down*. Then one day Harold flipped through mom's word-search puzzle book and discovered random letters circled rather than actual words. I stared in stunned silence as he pointed out her handiwork to me. I grabbed the newspaper and turned to the crossword puzzle she had completed earlier. More gibberish. Completely unnerved, I couldn't think of a single believable excuse to rationalize it in my mind. At the same time, I had no idea what to do about it. The revelation paralyzed me. While mentally coming to grips with the situation and trying to figure out a proper course of action, another troubling change was occurring right under my nose.

For years, each afternoon, when I came home from teaching my eighth-graders, mom would joke about the wayward teenagers in my charge, "So, what kind of trouble did they get in today?" I enjoyed sharing the ups and downs of my job with her, while we slurped our fruit smoothies together. We'd laugh about the crazy antics of my students or the unrealistic expectations of the school district. Without my mother actually saying it, I could tell she was proud of me and admired my work with the kids.

Over the course of only a few weeks, I watched her enthusiastic interest turn into blank stares and random statements such as, "The windows are dirty." I found it infuriating at first (even though the windows were indeed dirty!). *Why is mom talking about the windows? Why doesn't she pay attention?*

Initially, I didn't consider my mother's inane comments to be as bizarre as you might think. For most of my adult life, I had usually found her conversation to be somewhat unsatisfying because mom never had any real news of her own to share. Jinx had no outside interests or friends and she rarely left the house, since she didn't drive. She held no political opinions, nor knowledge of world events because it's hard to glean much from

27

reading only newspaper headlines, the comics, and Dear Abby. Consequently, when we conversed, I did most of the talking.

The alarming new change I observed in my mother's communication disturbed me much more because her responses came way out of left field and bore no relevance to what I was saying to her. Every time I tried to converse with mom now, her replies became increasingly disconnected. I soon realized a meaningful dialogue with her was futile. I felt as if I were talking to a young child...because I *finally* realized, I kind of was.

The sad truth was impossible to deny: Mom could no longer process my words, which meant she could no longer understand them. Which also meant she couldn't possibly reply accordingly. Instead of conversing on topic, she made random statements like, "It looks windy outside," or asked unrelated questions such as, "Is Harold still at work?" My mother had lost her ability to participate in the natural exchange of thoughts and feelings necessary for conversation.

A heavy wave of profound loss washed over me, as the full scope of that painful realization sank in. The expression of our words and our ideas is fundamentally who we are. Mom's was apparently gone for good now – which meant a large part of her was too. Our spirited talks after work would *never again* be a part of my day. Then the guilt set in. I had always longed for more interesting and stimulating conversation with my mother. Why couldn't I have appreciated the charm and simplicity of her company? Now I would have nothing. The depth of my self-anger and remorse physically sickened me. I already missed her.

It was finally the awakening I needed to understand and admit my mother's mental condition went WAY beyond the common forgetfulness of old age – and it had for many months. However, my reluctance to accept it had nothing to do with the usual shame or embarrassment often derived from a loved one's dementia; such stigma had actually never occurred to me. I think, perhaps, my blindness partially stemmed from my mother's mastery at concealing any weakness or vulnerability she had throughout her life, resulting in my brain's refusal to see her that way – as either weak or vulnerable. That blindness had prevented me from objectively assessing the observable facts and recognizing the heartbreaking truth of her cognitive decline.

I said it aloud to myself for the first time, "Mom has dementia."

The 7 Stages of Alzheimer's Disease

Stage 1: No Impairment
- No symptoms of dementia are evident

Stage 2: Very Mild Decline
- Undistinguishable from normal age-related memory loss
- Losing things around the house

Stage 3: Mild Decline
- Difficulty remembering names, organizing/planning, finding the right word

Stage 4: Moderate Decline
- Clear-cut Alzheimer symptoms
- Difficulty doing simple arithmetic
- Inability to manage finances/pay bills
- Poor short-term memory (can't remember what they had for lunch)

Stage 5: Moderate Severe Decline
- Needs help with day-to-day activities
- Significant confusion
- Difficulty dressing properly
- Hard to recall simple details of life
- Maintains functionality – still able to bathe and toilet independently

Stage 6: Severe Decline
- Needs constant supervision and frequently requires professional care
- Loss of bladder and bowel control
- Wandering
- Unawareness/confusion regarding surroundings
- Needs help toileting and bathing

Stage 7: Very Severe Decline
- Nearing death
- May lose ability to swallow
- Needs assistance for daily living
- No insight into their condition
- Lose ability to communicate or respond to environment

**According to Alzheimers.net, affiliated with "A Place for Mom, Inc."

APPREHENSION & RESENTMENT

I'm embarrassed to admit, by the time I finally pulled my head out of the sands of denial and acknowledged my mother's true mental state, she was probably already at stage five Alzheimer's; moderate to severe cognitive decline. Hindsight is always 20/20. But moving forward, one truth could not be disputed; Jinx would be needing intensive long-term care.

People often ask me, "How did YOU end up caring for your mom, Marlene? What made you take that on, instead of putting her in a memory-care facility?"

Believe me, I did a lot of deep soul-searching before ultimately accepting the job of primary caregiver to my mother. I knew as her dementia progressed, we would eventually be switching roles with each other; I'd become her parent and she, my child – just like in both *Freaky Friday* movies – where the mother and daughter must learn to empathize and understand each other. Except *unlike* in the films, any new insight could only come from me. Not fair! Of course, I soon realized there was nothing fair about *any* of this dementia stuff.

How do you set aside countless nagging childhood issues in order to selflessly care for a parent who is becoming increasingly dependent on you? It's impossible to merely stow a lifetime of emotional baggage in a temporary cargo area. Of Jinx's four children, I was the only one who didn't view her through rose-colored glasses. My siblings placed her on an idealistic pedestal, and to this day, defend her every past action. But many

31

of my issues ran deep and personal growth doesn't happen overnight. I still had a couple of dinosaur-size bones to pick with her.

Twenty years earlier, when Jinx initially moved in with us, I had accepted the idea of taking care of her, *someday*, to some degree. Since mom was only 67-years-old then, that was a distant and abstract notion. Plus, she had enjoyed such robust health her entire life, I foolishly imagined it continuing well into her nineties and ending with mom peacefully dying in her sleep. The possibility of having to care for an Alzheimer's patient NEVER entered my mind.

Now it seemed, I was presumably the *default* caregiver, by virtue of mom living in my home. Nobody ever told me the phrase "possession is 9/10 of the law" pertained to the ownership of people. The situation put me to mind of when baby Caitlin needed her diaper changed, and Harold and I employed the "finders-keepers" rule.

The circumstances of how Jinx came to live with us are highly unusual. Believe it or not, the invitation came not from me – but from her son-in-law. I know I should've considered myself lucky to have such a caring, empathetic spouse, but I sure didn't see it that way at the time. It was six years after my father died, and we were only twenty-eight-years-old, when Harold made the following offer to mom, without consulting me.

"Jinx, you shouldn't have to live all by yourself. When we move back to Arizona and build our house in Fountain Hills, we'll add a bedroom and bathroom on for you and you can move in with us."

Excuse me? What man (who values his life) does that? His proposal sparked an argument lasting the entire six-hour drive back to our home in California.

"Why didn't you ask me first? Maybe I don't want to live with my mother!"

"I didn't think you'd mind, since she's your mom. I figured you'd want to help her."

Ouch. Way to shame me, Harold!

The truth was, I didn't feel like living with mom *again*, so soon. We had already come to her rescue five years earlier.

Upon daddy's passing, mom found herself in serious financial straits; my parents had made some unfortunate financial miscalculations. She wasn't yet old enough to collect Social Security, and her only means of support was from babysitting kids, plus contributions from Jaime, who still lived at home.

Harold and I stepped in to help her for one year. We rented out our own house – bearing a fifty-dollar-a-month loss – and moved in with mom, paying her mortgage and utilities. Even during the 1980's (when it was easier for young people to get ahead), that was not a typical thing for twenty-three-year-olds to do. When the year was over, Harold and I moved to California, and soon afterward, Jaime got married, which left Jinx on her own.

The prospect of living with my mother again did not become appealing until Caitlin was born, when suddenly, having a built-in, babysitter grandma sounded like a fair trade. In 1993, the four of us moved into our new house together.

Our multi-generational household worked out exceptionally well for everybody and we never regretted the decision to include mom. Ours was a uniquely peaceful and mutually beneficial living arrangement. I credit much of our familial harmony to Jinx's wisdom and discipline. Having endured a meddling mother-in-law herself, mom vowed never to be one, actually proclaiming to me, "You rule the roost now!" She meant it and she lived by it every day.

If only my mother would have at least *tried* to make a life for herself. But she hadn't. The only time she left the house was when one of my siblings, usually Karen, took her out – about three Sundays per month. That was the extent of Jinx's social life. Even when Caitlin had a sleepover at a friend's house, Harold and I still never had the place to ourselves, to enjoy as a couple. My annoyance and disgust soon snowballed. I used to refer to mom as "the potted plant," because she appeared to have taken root in the family room couch. Our home may have been free from discord, but I harbored some festering issues. I resented sacrificing my solitude and privacy.

Consequently, I had to ask myself, "If *that* insignificant level of sacrifice bothers you, how in the world can you even consider the role of mom's caregiver?" There were so many formidable unknowns:

- How many years would mom need care?
- How bad would her dementia get?
- What about Harold and Caitlin?
- What would our lives be like?

And that was only the tip of the iceberg – the tiny part I could see – sticking out of the water. I knew there also had to be a more daunting mass looming below the surface as well; questions I couldn't conceive of yet.

The three of us had hectic lives. Harold ran his own construction business, Caitlin worked and went to college, and I was a teacher. How would we manage mom's care while we were at work, especially as it became more burdensome and time intensive? I didn't have the answers, but I was sure of one very comforting thing. My husband and daughter would fully support me if I chose to care for mom in our home.

All cards on the table, I resented the prospect of interrupting our lives to ensure mom's welfare *again*. Sometimes it gets tiring wearing the mantel of "problem solver." My siblings had a variety of financial and family hardships which precluded them from taking care of our mother. The reality was if I didn't do it, she would have to be placed in a memory-care facility. End of story. How could I live with that guilt when I knew my family and I were perfectly capable of doing the job?

As I began contemplating the enormous commitment involved in the selfless task of caregiving, a myriad of sticky issues regarding my mother began to rear their heads. Perhaps, I was trying to rationalize why bailing on mom would be a perfectly acceptable thing to do. I had discarded most of the trivial childhood grievances along the path to adulthood, but others had been stewing for many years – resulting in some tough to chew meat.

First and foremost on my list of unresolved anger was the appalling way my mother "threw in the towel" after my dad's death. Fifteen years after his passing, while trying to persuade her to visit the senior center in town, she flat out refused, citing the excuse, "When daddy died, my life ended too." Mom was only 56 when she became a widow! Her negative outlook infuriated me. I still can't imagine having such a mindset, at so young an age.

It's disheartening watching a physically healthy parent do little else besides sit on a couch for over thirty years because they've deemed their "life is over." Especially when they have at least a dozen people – their children and their spouses, plus grandchildren – who cherish them. It offended and insulted me, on a personal level. In her 32 years as a widow, Jinx could have enjoyed a full life – even a couple more husbands. I wholeheartedly believe my dad would have remarried under the same circumstances.

The indignance I held for my mother's defeatist attitude left me with a difficult question to reconcile. Why should I give up God only knows how many years of my life taking care of an individual who has lost the will to live?

Also high on the list of sore points: The superficial nature of our mother-daughter relationship. For as long as I could remember, I ached for us to be closer. I longed to know my mother – as a woman and as a person. What were her hopes, dreams, and goals? Her concerns, frustrations, disappointments, and regrets? I really didn't know because she never shared those thoughts with me. She was so damn private. We never had deep talks. But I wouldn't say she was a totally closed book; more like a children's picture book – pretty illustrations with few words.

Even after twenty years of living under the same roof – with mom being an integral part of our lives – something still prevented me from feeling *truly close* to her. An unspoken, intangible barrier existed between us; one I believe she probably erected as a new mother, while defining her parent/child boundaries.

When it came to kids, Jinx did not see them as people in their own right, worthy of respect; respect was reserved for adults only. The feelings and opinions of children carried no weight and held no value. I often heard the words, "You're not a grown-up – nobody listens to you, or cares what you have to say." Talking back, sulking, using a "snotty tone," or questioning her too severely were grounds for a slap or an all-out spanking. It was far better to zip your lip. The status quo continued unchanged into my teen years.

As I entered adulthood, I figured at some point I'd rise to her equal in her eyes; mom's guard would come down, and we'd meld into best buds. I pictured the two of us sharing a chummy exchange of "girl talk" over coffee. But I waited in vain. She was the mother and I was the daughter. We were never friends. The wall between us remained steadfast.

It was then I made a conscious decision to shut down honest communication with her. *If she won't open up to me, I won't confide in her either. So there!* During those years, regarding my aloofness, mom used to say, "Still waters run deep. I don't know who you are." And I would deliberately ignore her comment – reinforcing my mother's barrier with steel bars of my own.

Another hindrance to my relationship with mom was her seriously outdated views, which she forced upon me and which I bitterly resented. I didn't want to be her "Mini-Me." I remember being at odds with my mother for much of my childhood because she controlled every aspect of my life. I couldn't wait to reach adulthood, so I could be myself.

To me, mom was like an alien from another planet or a lost time traveler from the 1940s. She had no notion of contemporary ideas, styles, or culture. She reminded me of Rip Van Winkle! I understand she was raised during a different era, but at some point a person has to acknowledge the world has changed. Jinx was stuck in a time warp – specifically one filled with Shirley Temple movies. This wouldn't have bothered me so much if she hadn't inflicted it upon me. She didn't care that the tap dancing moppet had no relevance in my 1960s, flower-power world.

In an effort to create her own personal Shirley, Mom started perming my naturally straight hair when I was three-years-old! She styled it daily with Dippity-do (remember that stuff?), in old-fashioned "bologna curls," all the way up to age twelve. Frilly dresses, ankle socks and patent leather Mary Janes completed my ridiculous *Rebecca of Sunnybrook Farm* ensemble. I had zero say in my own appearance. Surrounded by a school full of "Marcia Bradys," I felt like a circus freak.

Besides my hair and clothes, my mother apparently also felt my own body was none of my business either. She saw no reason to inform me my

37

anatomy included a vagina. Only a minor detail! I was not privy to that information until age ten, when my fifth grade teacher sent the "Your Changing Body" booklets home. Imagine my surprise! I have to assume mom considered female genitalia to be an entirely sexual matter, reserved for a special "unveiling" at first menstruation. Why bother telling your daughter she has a vagina when you can conveniently describe childbirth as, "Babies come out of the mama's behind like poop." This ludicrous explanation resulted in vivid nightmares, where I helplessly watched my newborn infant get sucked down the swirling water of our toilet.

During my high school years (circa 1976), mom preached a litany of archaic ideas to me. Here are my top five favorites, in no particular order:

1. Science and math are for boys. You don't need to care about those subjects.
2. Tampons are for married women only. You can "break yourself," and if you do, no man will ever want you because you'll be "used goods."
3. You don't need a college education, since you're going to be financially supported by your husband.
4. Sex is dirty, for an unmarried woman. For a wife, it's beautiful. If you get divorced, it's dirty again.
5. A bride must give her husband the "gift" of her virginity on the wedding night.* *Grooms did not have to reciprocate. Men got a free pass on sexual morality because "they have their needs." Presumably, mom believed women had no such needs. Premarital sex privileges were granted to my brothers based on this premise.

All of these ridiculous notions culminated in a final earth-shattering crescendo, the summer after high school graduation. Harold Jackson (whom I dated my entire senior year) and I had set money aside to take a month-long road trip to Canada and around the western states. Our departure date was set for July 21, 1978. Only ten days prior, I nervously dropped the bomb on my folks.

Daddy had openly disapproved of my barefoot, "hippie boyfriend" – the one with the goatee, long hair, killer abs, and worst of all, HIS OWN APARTMENT. My parent's response to my trip announcement? Instant disownment if I "honeymooned" without benefit of marriage. Traveling together while engaged was also not an option because of the "used goods" problem. God forbid we broke up during the trip, and Harold cast me aside before saying, "I do." What man would have me then?

I blame my father more than my mother in this particular case, since he cast the most repudiation and shame upon me. But mom stood in solidarity with him, so I held her equally culpable for forcing me to marry at the childish age of 18. Both my parents knew it was not in my best interest, but they put my back to the wall, hoping we would nix the trip altogether. Instead, their stubborn daughter decided to spitefully move ahead with wedding plans, in a manner they deemed "flippant and farcical."

In one week, Harold and I made arrangements to be married, and July 21, 1978 became our wedding day. The bride wore her prom dress, and the groom bought new corduroy Levi's for the occasion. Afterward, I handed my parents the marriage certificate – my way of showing them it meant nothing to me – and drove away with Harold in his pickup truck on our intended trip.

My dad eventually warmed to my new husband – once Harold cut his hair. I wish my father would have lived long enough to fully appreciate the truly amazing man my "hippie boyfriend" turned out to be; the stellar "papa" who raised an extraordinary daughter, and the selfless son-in-law who lovingly cared for Jinx for over twenty years.

Ultimately, my gnawing ambivalence about committing to mom's long-term care led to a final examination of my reasonable and well-founded objections:

- Harold and I had already devoted more than our share of years ensuring mom's well-being
- Jinx had, long ago, lost her enthusiasm for living
- Our mother-daughter relationship lacked an intimate bond and we had virtually nothing in common
- My mother's controlling parenting had left me bereft of something everybody needs from a parent – *unconditional acceptability*

Oftentimes, judgements such as mine – disrespect for a person's ideas and life choices – goes hand-in-hand with disrespect for the individual as well. And that's when the fundamental distinction hit me. Despite our *enormous* differences and my many unresolved issues, my immense respect for my mother had never faltered. In fact, I couldn't think of anything she *ever* did that brought shame or disrespect upon her. Jinx Scribner had led a simple life of grace, humility and gratitude. I was proud to call her my mother.

The bottom line came down to this: Through the years, mom had helped Harold, Caitlin, and me much as we had helped her. If *she* hadn't earned our care, nobody had. Besides, truth be told, my own daughter probably would have sooner put me in a home, than her beloved grandmother.

WHY HER?

The average age, at *diagnosis* of Alzheimer's disease, is 80. Mom's dementia symptoms began manifesting a few months after her 81st birthday. Prior to that, she had always been quite healthy. Amazingly, the only daily prescription she took was her thyroid medicine. I had to ask myself, "Why her?" I wondered what had caused the deterioration of her brain. Her genes? Her lifestyle choices? Her advanced age? Or was it a combination of things? Could she have done anything to avoid it? Did she simply live too damn long? Another question I had was why dementia is becoming increasingly prevalent globally? Over 60 million people worldwide currently have a dementia-related disease.

The word dementia terrified me. It conjured up images of insanity and mental institutions; of people losing their minds; of my mother losing *her* mind. It's hard to process the idea of your parent having *progressive, permanent brain failure*. I wondered if mom's dementia automatically meant she had Alzheimer's disease because I honestly did not know. I had heard the terms used interchangeably, but upon researching them both, I learned they are not the same.

Speaking of research, we are lucky to live in a time where we have, literally, a wealth of information at our fingertips. The medical and scientific findings in this chapter were culled from websites, conferences, publications, and seminars from the following: Alzheimer's Association,

Alzheimer's Foundation of America, MedlinePlus, Caregiver Homes, Mayo Clinic News Network, WebMD, Healthline, and AARP.

Dementia should not be used synonymously with Alzheimer's. It's a general "umbrella term" for progressive, neurobiological disorders encompassing a group of symptoms impacting mental tasks like reasoning, communication ability, behavior, and memory. Alzheimer's is one type of dementia and the most common. A person with Alzheimer's has dementia, but a person with dementia does not necessarily have Alzheimer's.

Senility is a term once used to describe all forms of dementia, but it's no longer used as a diagnosis. A person can have more than one type of dementia simultaneously, and it can be triggered by other diseases such as Parkinson's and Huntington's disease. Here are a few other types of dementia and their symptoms:

- **Frontotemporal Dementia (FTD)** – Loss of empathy, inappropriate inhibition, & apathy
- **Lewy Body Dementia (LBD)** – Confusion, rigid muscles, hallucinations, balance issues, shuffling walk, & memory loss
- **Huntington's Disease Dementia (HD)** – Anger, trouble speaking clearly, jerky body movements, & difficulty walking
- **Parkinson's Disease Dementia (PD)** – Tremors, impaired balance, memory loss, & diminished attention span

Neurodegeneration – the destruction of brain cells (neurons) – is the leading biological cause of dementia. There are other forms of dementia which result from mini-strokes, traumatic brain injury, and even infections like Mad Cow Disease, but I prefer to focus on the type my mother had – Alzheimer's. Individuals with Alzheimer's disease experience the slow, progressive death of brain cells and a total shrinkage in brain size, which leaves them with fewer nerve cells and less connections. Brain cells are not repairable and there is no cure. Changes in the brain, typical of Alzheimer's, can occur *twenty-five years* before symptoms appear.

What types of brain changes actually destroy the neurons? They read like a science textbook:

- Amyloid plaques (sticky barnacle-like proteins) interfering with connections and messages
- Tau deposits (twisted protein threads) clogging vital memory regions
- Tangled neurons (disrupting critical signals)
- Loss of glutamate (a major neurotransmitter)

But the key question everybody wants a definitive answer to is this: Why do some people live long lives without destructive brain changes, while others end up with dementia?

Despite decades of research, science has failed to provide a conclusive answer for *exactly* what triggers such complete devastation of the brain *or* to find a drug that can consistently alter the progression.

So, what *is* fueling the Alzheimer epidemic? For starters, Baby Boomers are aging into the range for dementia. Equally significant, is the undeniable trend of people living longer than ever before. The aging brain has more brain cell destruction, so the longer you live, the higher your chances are of getting the disease. When we look around, we see "eighty-somethings" everywhere. Nonagenarians, the folks who live into their 90's, are also becoming quite common. Beloved entertainers like Dick Van Dyke, Betty White, and Tony Bennett have been able to maintain not only razor-sharp minds, but also their immensely successful careers, proving advanced age is obviously not the only factor. Sadly, for far too many other individuals, their brains don't seem to be as resilient.

43

Another notable factor driving the epidemic is Type 2 diabetes. Researchers have known for many years that being overweight and having Type 2 diabetes increases the risk for developing Alzheimer's disease. Over time, diabetes can damage blood vessels in the brain. More recent discussions have now turned to Type 3 diabetes; a term proposed in research studies to classify Alzheimer's as a possible type of diabetes.

Type 3 diabetes occurs when neurons in the brain become unable to respond to insulin, which is necessary for essential tasks like learning and memory. The Alzheimer's gene (APOE4) can interrupt how the brain processes insulin. The gene plus the insulin resistance, caused by a high-fat diet, together induces insulin resistance in the brain. Alzheimer's appears to be another potential side-effect of the sugary, fatty, western-style diet.

Jinx did not have diabetes, nor was she ever overweight, but she definitely had a high-fat, high-sugar diet. The more I examined the possible risk factors for Alzheimer's, the more I realized how most of them are attributed to lifestyle choices. My mother seemed to be cooking up a perfect recipe for acquiring dementia for most of her life. Mom had MANY strikes against her. The following is a generally medically agreed upon list of culprits linked to Alzheimer's:

Links to Alzheimer's

- Chronic Stress & Depression
- Lack of Exercise
- Concussions
- Genetics
- Heart Disease
- Lack of Restorative Sleep
- Lack of Social Connection & Mental Stimulation
- Low Kidney Function
- High Blood Pressure
- Poor Nutrition
- Insulin Resistance & Diabetes
- Inflammation from Toxins & Infection

Yikes! Mom had about 75% of the items on the list! She did not have low kidney function or any concussions, but let's take a look at the other factors.

Poor Nutrition: A quick inventory of Jinx's diet compared with recommended brain health foods suggests mom made abominable food choices.

Recommended "Brainpower" Diet	Jinx's Comparable Diet
Leafy Greens (Kale, Spinach)	Iceberg Lettuce
Cruciferous Veggies (Brussel Sprouts, Cauliflower)	Canned Corn
Whole Grains (Quinoa, 100% Wheat Bread)	White Bread and Rice Cereal
Berries and Cherries	Canned Peaches in Heavy Syrup and Grape Jelly
Beans and Legumes (Kidney, Pinto)	Canned Pork 'n' Beans
Omega-3 Fats (Salmon, Tuna)	No Fish Ever!
Raw Unsalted Nuts (Almonds, Walnuts)	Snicker's Candy Bars
Lean Meat (Chicken, Turkey)	Beef Hot Dogs and Bologna
Tomatoes, Beets, Asparagus, and Carrots	Huzzah! She Actually Ate Those

Insulin Resistance and Diabetes: Jinx was not diabetic, but she had a sizable sweet tooth. Not only during her senior years when taste buds diminish — but her whole life. Mom had always been quite the connoisseur of Popsicles, Nilla Wafers, Ginger Snaps, cinnamon graham crackers and gumdrops. Her diet contained high amounts of sugar, carbohydrates, nitrates, and processed/prepackaged foods. In short, mom ate a lot of crap!

45

It's amazing she lived as long as she did. She obviously ate whatever she liked, with no concern for nutrition or health.

How Jinx was able to maintain her trim figure throughout the years, with those abysmal eating habits, is another mystery. I suspect since she was more than halfway through her life before high fructose corn syrup, hybrid wheat, and trans-fat infiltrated our national food supply, it most likely helped shield her from the rampant obesity so prevalent today. She was also fairly physically active for most of her life.

Lack of Exercise: Mom didn't lift weights or attend aerobic classes, but she was no stranger to good, old-fashioned exercise. Working around the house and yard kept her remarkably fit, trim, and healthy. She maintained a weight of about 130 lbs. on her 5'4" frame well into her 60's. I'll never forget, how at age 70, she energetically helped shovel a truckload of gravel around our yard. My mother could always be counted on to enthusiastically join us in landscaping our Arizona desert property, be it preparing flower beds, trimming hedges, or even digging holes for trees.

A few years after we were married, my always forthright husband confessed to having "sized-up" my mother's figure during our courtship.

"I checked out Jinx, to get an idea of how *you* might age," Harold admitted to me, out of the blue. "She looked great for a woman in her fifties. I didn't see any weird veins sticking out of her legs, or cellulite, or stretch marks. Nothing sagged, she was slim, and she still looked good in shorts! I figured you'd probably be the same way."

Sadly, during the decade leading up to her dementia symptoms, mom got virtually no exercise. She became extremely sedentary, spending most of her time on the couch.

Inflammation from Toxins: My mother never smoked, but she did breathe in my father's second-hand, cigarette smoke for about 30 years, until he quit in 1976. Who knows how much those toxins affected her health. She also had exposure to asbestos in the factory she worked in for a couple years as a teenager.

High Blood Pressure and Heart Disease: As far as high blood pressure and heart disease are concerned, mom was not diagnosed with either condition until the last 18 months of her life.

Chronic Stress and Depression: Jinx probably suffered from depression. Her husband's premature and unexpected death — at age fifty-eight from arteriosclerosis — certainly triggered trauma, stress, and long-lasting despair. I don't think mom ever fully recovered from it. She never dated again or displayed the slightest interest in any other men. Not wanting anyone to feel sorry for her, she wore her usual cheery smile, and kept much of her grief to herself. With the exception of a short-term Valium prescription when daddy died, mom took nothing for anxiety, sleep, pain, or depression, and never drank alcohol. She faced each day with a clear, unaltered mental state, but I had to wonder what was really going on behind her brave face.

Lack of Social Connection and Mental Stimulation: One thing most medical experts agree on is the importance of keeping the mind active in order to maintain memory, concentration, and problem-solving ability. Working out our mental muscles is as necessary as daily physical exercise in the fight against dementia, and the phrase "use it or lose it" applies every bit as much to our cognitive ability as it does the rest of our physiology.

Challenging ourselves mentally is critical to keeping our minds sharp; preferably via activities stimulating enough to keep our neurotransmitters firing. Learning a foreign language or a musical instrument, traveling to new places, taking college courses, or engaging in creative endeavors are all beneficial. Equally important is staying active socially and conversing with other people. Sad to say, even before she became a widow, my mother did NONE of those things, which made any depression she might have developed afterward harder to detect

Challenging her mind and learning new things never interested mom. I believe it actually made her downright uncomfortable. My repeated promptings to meet new people or do anything remotely social were shot down at every turn. The town we live in has a large number of active retirees, and the nearby senior center offers a wide variety of activities such as cards, jazzercise, quilting groups, and watercolor painting. Mom always refused to go. During the twenty years she lived in Fountain Hills with us, I didn't make the slightest dent in her resolve to remain isolated within our friendly community.

Genetics: See the following chapter (Jinx's Folks).

Lack of Restorative Sleep: I didn't know my mother suffered from a lack of restorative sleep until her dementia symptoms were already in full bloom. Turns out, she had severely disrupted sleep patterns, which is a significant risk factor. While we sleep, our brains perform vital work; cleaning out toxins, storing what we learn, making connections, and combining memories. When sleep is denied, we end up with one big jumbled, dysfunctional mess in our heads.

Approximately two years into Jinx's symptoms, a neurologist referred her for an overnight stay in a hospital to have a sleep-study performed. It revealed mom had obstructive sleep apnea (OSA), which interrupted her breathing an average of 50 times EACH HOUR. That's almost every minute! It was one of the worst cases the doctor had ever seen! Throughout the night, her tongue continuously dropped back and obstructed her airway, which also caused her heavy snoring. I wondered when her tongue first started blocking her breathing to that extent, since bulldozer noises had been penetrating her bedroom walls the entire two decades she lived with us.

The doctor recommended a CPAP (Continuous Positive Airway Pressure) machine for mom to use at night to keep her tongue in place and the airway open. The large, plastic mask fit over her nose and mouth, similar to one used for oxygen, and connected to a laptop-size air-pressure machine, via a hose. The device was supposed to provide a continuous flow of air to her all night long, thus ensuring a sound, restful night's sleep.

Incredibly, the doctor failed to understand that Jinx's lack of cognitive function would render the CPAP an effort in futility. Since mom couldn't comprehend the need for the scary-looking device, it confused her and caused her great anxiety, which added undue stress to our bedtime routine. After much coercion, I would eventually strap the mask onto her face and she'd quickly doze off. Within two to three hours, however, my mother would get out of bed to use the bathroom, take off the mask, and leave it off. She couldn't have put it back on even if she had wanted to. By then, mom already lacked the mental and manual dexterity necessary to do so.

One night, she forgot to remove the mask when she got out of bed and because she was tethered to the machine – which was plugged into the wall – it jerked her backward with enough force to pull her to the floor. Thankfully, mom didn't injure herself, but it was the last time I forced her to wear the device.

Ultimately, I deemed the CPAP a complete waste of time and effort. Although the sleep study had correctly revealed a serious disruption in mom's sleep, it was too late in the game to determine whether it had caused her dementia – or to do anything about it.

Perhaps we'll never know the exact cause of Jinx's Alzheimer's, but new research is popping up all the time. The latest studies are showing a connection between brain health and oral health; specifically a link between the destruction of neurons and gingivitis. Imagine if preventing Alzheimer's is as simple as brushing your teeth. Incidentally (or not?), my mother wore upper dentures.

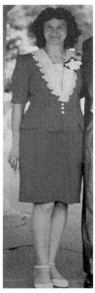

Mom, at Billy's wedding, 1994
At age 68, I'd say her genes look pretty great!

JINX'S FOLKS & GENETIC RISKS

Without question, Jinx had major risk factors for acquiring dementia, but what about her genetic predisposition? Even though it's on the list of causes, heredity really is in a category of its own. It's not about lifestyle choices or avoidable circumstances; we're all stuck with the genes we are handed at birth. I started wondering if Alzheimer's ran in my mother's family.

I confess to never having given the matter much consideration before, but if you had a grandfather who thought ABC (already-been-chewed) gum from the gutter was a safe treat for a child, and a grandmother who didn't visit a doctor until she had a fist-size hole in her chest, you *might* wonder if perhaps there was some mental problems floating around in the family.

Most people are probably aware Alzheimer's can be inherited. Approximately 20% of the general population has the dreaded gene, APOE4, and it's seen in more than half of all Alzheimer's cases, but prediction of the disease is still tricky. It's possible to receive the gene from one or both parents, but it doesn't *automatically* mean you'll get Alzheimer's. Conversely, not possessing the gene does not *preclude* you from getting it. Personally, I'd prefer not to know if I have the gene because I could waste valuable years of my life worrying needlessly. Since nobody in Jinx's family ever underwent DNA testing, there's no way to know with certainty if heredity played a part in her illness. All we can do is speculate.

I'm pleased to report that diving into her family gene pool was not the toilsome task I had imagined. Sure, it required a bit of digging into my relatives' health and causes of death, but it also afforded me a lighthearted stroll back in time with my dear grandparents.

My mother – Josephine Ann Klesik – was born on December 4, 1926, the fifth child of Polish immigrants, Anna and Joseph. Rumor has it, Joseph immigrated to the states illegally. The story, in a nutshell, handed down through the years goes as follows: Joseph and his brother tended the gardens around the royal palace of the King of Austria (Poland being part of the Austria-Hungary Empire at the time). The brother held immigration papers to come to America but changed his mind at the last minute, allowing Joseph to make the trip in his place. Such an occurrence would be impossible today.

Mom never told me how her parents met or when they wed, only that theirs was an arranged marriage; one actually *forced* upon her mother. When Joseph asked Anna's father for his daughter's hand, he enthusiastically agreed without consulting his daughter first, unaware Anna's heart belonged to another – an unnamed man whose photo she secretly kept for her entire life. Over time, Anna came to love Joseph and the marriage endured for more than 50 years.

Josephine was proud to be her "pop's" namesake. She had three sisters, Agnes, Margaret and Sophie, and a brother named Martin. Her parents' first-born child, a son, died shortly after birth. The family called Josephine "Josie" and to this day, every one of her nieces and nephews still refer to her as their "Aunt Josie."

A petite, spindly girl, with dark hair and almost black eyes, Josie grew up in a modest house in the tiny borough of Manville, New Jersey. By all accounts, she was a cheerful child who loved to draw, roller-skate, jump

52

rope, and play hopscotch. Her folks had no money for extras, so in her teen years, she started designing and sewing all her own clothes (yes, isn't that what we all do?).

The Klesiks were simple, working-class people. Anna stayed home and raised the five kids (along with rabbits and chickens for food), and Joseph worked at the neighborhood factory, Johns-Manville Corporation (aka J-M). The evenings were for family fun, when Joseph would entertain his wife and children with spirited music.

Before doing so, he'd summon one of the brood to fill his small, crystal glass with liquor. My mother loved it when it was her turn.

"Josie! I'll take my whiskey now!"

His obedient daughter would retrieve his shot of booze as quickly as she could and scurry back with it. Then he'd toss it down his gullet with gusto and commence playing on his wooden squeezebox or trusty fiddle. Polka dancing soon ensued around the living room.

My mother's favorite "pop story" involved her 8th grade graduation ceremony. It was one I'd heard dozens of times, but never grew tired of.

Josie and her classmates waited excitedly on the stage of the school gymnasium, listening for the principal to call their names. When Mr. Zorella finally announced, "Josephine Ann Klesik," she nervously strode toward him to accept her diploma, knowing her family's eyes were on her. Suddenly, she heard her pop's voice cry out from the audience as he leapt to his feet, wildly waving his hat and shouting in his Polish accent, "Datsah MY daughtah! Datsah MY Josie!"

Her pop hadn't embarrassed her at all. On the contrary, it was one of Josie's proudest moments. And I could still see it in mom's face every time she told the story.

My grandpa passed away in 1961, when I was only one-year-old, so I have no actual memories of him; only the lovely ones my mother instilled me. I wish I could have known him; he seemed like such an interesting fellow. Old photos of Joseph reveal a snappy dresser, always sporting a stylish fedora, a suit vest, and leather dress shoes. Karen, who had him in her life for thirteen years, told me he rolled his own cigarettes.

Now for the ABC gum. My sister also shared with me the curious tales of how grandpa would pick up filthy gum from the side of the road and offer it to her as a treat. Our mother had prewarned Karen not to accept any "gifts" from grandpa: If he gave her anything, she needed to show it to mom immediately. So when he gave her the ABC gum, she always handed it right over, like a good girl.

My sister has no further explanation about this! Hello? What the hell kind of story is that? Nobody questioned this behavior? Did grandpa chew used gum, himself? This didn't outrage my mother? If only I could interrogate her. I have to wonder if grandpa suffered from some form of dementia because that is truly a demented thing to do!

Two decades after my grandfather's death, Johns-Manville filed for bankruptcy under the weight of unprecedented asbestos injury claims. When I asked mom if her father had died of an asbestos-related illness, she stopped and to think about it for a minute before giving me the following unfathomable answer.

"Gosh, I don't know…maybe. Nobody said what happened – he just got sick. He never went to the doctor. Back then, when people died, no one asked why."

Joseph Klesik lived to be 72 years-old, which is relatively young by today's standards. Only three percent of people between ages 65 and 74 have Alzheimer's. He didn't live long enough to find out if Alzheimer's lurked within and nobody questioned his demise. My money is on death by ABC gum.

My grandma passed away when I was nine – certainly old enough to have vivid memories – but all mine of her are hazy, and oddly, in black and white. Perhaps, because most photos of grandma are too. I remember her as a kind, patient, round-bodied woman, with a gentle smile; one who resembled the stereotypical grandmother of the era in her housedress, apron, hairnet, and thick stockings rolled down to the knees. My family referred to her as "Little Grandma," only to distinguish her from my dad's mother – aka "Big Grandma." Both women were tiny, only 5 feet in height, but Big Grandma was thin, so she looked taller.

Although Anna Klesik wasn't as rambunctious as her husband, she was pretty darn bold in her own right, especially for a young mother of five in the 1930s. The stories my mother told me about her seemed entirely out of character for the normally stoic and religious grandmother I knew. On more than one occasion in church, Anna became quite upset with the parish priest.

It seems Father John had scolded his flock one Sunday for not opening their hearts (and wallets) wide enough.

"I don't want to see pennies in the collection basket!" he railed from the pulpit.

Upon hearing the announcement, Anna fumed quietly in the pew, "Fine! You don't want my pennies? I don't give you nutting den!"

On a different sabbath, Father John's sermon to the congregation rubbed Anna the wrong way once again, when he relayed the Pope's latest decree.

"All good Catholics must keep multiplying if they expect eternal life in heaven with the Lord."

Young Josie heard her mother mumble angrily under her breath, "Oh yeah? Is da Pope gonna feed all my kids too? I don't t'ink so!"

Definitely a spunky woman! But my all-time favorite story about my grandmother is when she took her own husband to court. I don't know if she had any children yet, but at some point early in her marriage, her hubby decided he wasn't going to work anymore. He told Anna SHE needed to take a job instead. Astoundingly, my Little Grandma brought him before a local judge who ruled in her favor and severely berated him.

"Joseph Klesik, you are in the United States of America now. Here, it is the man's job to work. In this country, if you don't work, you go to jail!"

The judge's threat was enough to make Joseph obey the law for the remainder of their marriage.

Unfortunately, my grandmother was not wise about everything. She allowed Josie to drop out of high school her junior year. When her daughter asked her for a new bicycle Anna replied, "It's too much money. If you want a new bike, go to work and buy one yourself." So Josie dropped out and went to work at the J-M factory (exposing her to toxic carcinogens). It's still hard for me to believe my mother quit school to buy herself a bicycle! I presume that must have been a common and reasonable thing to do in 1940's wartime America.

Strangely, I have no memories of Little Grandma visiting our home. My dad always dropped us off at her place – similar to church. Her house was *way* better than church though. She always had her signature snack – pumpernickel rye bread slices sprinkled liberally with sugar – waiting for us. And she had the best toys in her closet, including a beautiful life-size doll I coveted for my own.

Anna Klesik passed away of breast cancer on Memorial Day, 1969. That's where the unimaginable hole in the chest comes in. My mom's account of her own mother's cancer diagnosis was relayed to me many times.

"By the time we took her to see a doctor, it was too late. I was in the examining room when she removed her slip – by then she had a fist-sized hole in her breast. I almost fainted from the horrible sight."

Anna had an irrational aversion to doctors, to the point of enduring agonizing pain. That mindset is crazy to most of us. She spent the final two years of her life bedridden, ravaged by the disease.

Little Grandma died at age 75, again, below the average age for acquiring Alzheimer's. While researching the deaths of my mother's siblings, I discovered all but one had passed away before age 80. One sister died of Diabetes at age 69; another from Mesothelioma Cancer (asbestos from J-M) at age 78; and her brother at age 67, from liver disease. The eldest sister succumbed to congestive heart failure, at age 85.

My aunt, who died at the young age of 69, also did so needlessly. Her doctor diagnosed her as diabetic, but she disagreed with his assessment and ignored it. "Doctors don't know everything," she proclaimed.

In conclusion, as far as I can tell, none of Jinx's immediate family members had Alzheimer's, but a few of them appeared to suffer from other serious mental ailments – namely ignorance and pigheadedness. If there are genes associated with those conditions, my mother definitely inherited them. She was another Klesik who avoided doctors. She stubbornly refused to have a medical check-up or physical exam from 1962 (the birth of her last child) to 1992 (until I dragged her to one). Her ridiculous reason being, "Why should I go to a doctor if I'm not sick?"

I have a better question: How can two sisters, who witnessed the unbearable – but avoidable – suffering and death of their own mother, follow the exact same path with their own health?

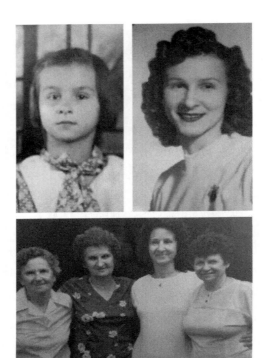

Upper Photos: *Young Josephine*
Bottom: *Josie & her three sisters*
(She's the tallest at 5'4")

PLAN OF ACTION

When I finally accepted my new role as mom's caregiver, I realized I had some urgent work to do on her behalf. Jinx's deteriorating mental state called for the serious formulation of a coherent, long-range plan of attack. But before I could give it one-hundred percent of my full concentration, I had to allow myself a day of quiet contemplation to cry and grieve the loss of my mother, as I knew her. The person I relied upon my whole life, to always be there for me, and care for me in any way she could, was slipping away – little by little – right in front of me. Although I had no idea what type of dementia she had, one thing was a certainty; her cognitive function was only going to get worse.

Once I had the mental clarity and composure to do so, I identified two areas of concern which warranted my immediate attention:

1. Has she been taking her daily thyroid pill? Does she even have any?
2. Has she been paying her bills? Is she financially secure?

Up until then, my involvement in those matters had been minimal. I didn't oversee my mother's medical or financial affairs. I took her to her regular doctor visits, but she handled her prescription refills. As far as her money was concerned, once a month I drove her to the bank, and all of her accounts were in both our names. Jinx had always managed her own money and health decisions, but I was reasonably certain such things were now beyond her capabilities, and I would need to take the helm.

Both subjects seemed kind of touchy to me. After all, what person wants to admit they're mentally slipping to the point they need their child to step in and handle their personal business? How could she not resent my interference? What excuse could I give my *extremely* private mother for rifling through her medicine cabinet, dresser drawers, purse, checkbook, wallet, and bank statements? She had only two rooms in the house which were solely hers, and I planned on turning them inside out. If she were guarding any secrets, I would surely uncover them. My investigation would undoubtedly arouse mom's suspicion and cause her to feel violated.

I had to laugh at the irony of the situation. Mom never guarded *anybody else's* secret. Au contraire, she delighted in spilling the beans! Jinx should have hung a "spoiler-alert" sign around her neck; every time she came home from the movies, she'd blurt out the ending.

"How was the movie, Ma? Did you like it?"

"Oh sure. The guy dies at the end, but it was still good."

One Christmas morning, Karen (who was 40 at the time) had a huge surprise for the family. She told us to wait on the sidewalk in front of mom's house. As we stood on the curb, wondering what the surprise could be, mom announced, "Karen got her license. She's gonna come driving down the street any minute!"

I don't know why my mother felt that was an acceptable thing to do. When I asked her why she spoiled the surprise, she said, "You were going to find out anyway." That was about twenty years *before* she got dementia and lost her social filter. The day I took a home pregnancy test and it turned out positive, I excitedly called mom with the news, but swore her to a temporary secrecy. As soon as I hung up the phone, I knew she was probably already dialing Karen!

Mom's own lack of discretion aside, I still felt weird about rooting through her private stuff. At first, I thought about asking Caitlin to take her

60

grandma out for a couple of hours, so I could freely snoop around. Upon further consideration, I decided to try a more honest and direct approach. Instead, I'd directly ask my mother's permission. I took the following tack (and it couldn't have been any easier):

"Mom, I was wondering if your thyroid medicine needs refilling. Is it okay if I take a look at the bottle? Where do you keep it?"

She looked up briefly from her puzzle book. "It's in my dresser. On top."

I found a half-dozen prescription bottles in the top drawer – all empty. The bottle with the most recent date on it, for a supply of thirty pills, was four months old. Also empty.

"I don't see any pills, Ma?" I yelled from her bedroom.

"They're in the big bottle," she shouted back. A moment later she appeared in the doorway. "See, right there." Mom pointed to the jar of chewable, calcium gummies setting on her dresser.

"These?" I picked up the bottle. "This is for calcium. What about your thyroid pills?"

She walked over and studied the bottle for a moment.

"Yeah, those. I take one every day."

I took several deep breaths as I stared at the calcium jar in disbelief and processed my mother's words. No further investigation was needed. I had my answer.

I smiled, despite the disconcerting realization. "I'm glad you've been taking your medicine, Ma."

"Oh, don't worry, I am!" she assured me. Then she sauntered out of the room, back to the couch and her puzzle book.

Oh shit! I had no idea what the possible medical repercussions might be for going three months without prescribed thyroid medicine. My next move was a call to her doctor for an immediate refill and an examination appointment. Already needing a mental break, I decided to put off the task of tackling mom's finances to the following day.

Convincing Jinx to give me carte blanche over her finances required no persuading at all – only the telling of a little white lie. I brought her into the study to show her my online bank account displayed on the screen of my laptop.

"Ma, the bank said everything is going to be computerized now. See, here's what mine looks like. They won't mail paper bank statements to you anymore. Have you ever used a computer?"

I knew my mother had never touched one in her life and had no desire to learn. Over the years, I had offered to show her how to email friends, surf the net, and play games like Scrabble, but she stubbornly refused every time.

"No, I don't do the computer."

"I can teach you if you want. It's not hard."

"Hell no! Not me!" She shook her head and laughed.

Like shooting fish in a barrel.

"Would it be easier if I pay your bills for you? You would still sign all the checks." (I could legally sign the checks myself, but I wanted to include her in the process.)

"Yeah, you won't steal my money. You're a nice girl." She playfully patted my head as if to say, "Good doggie."

Implementing my "plan of action" had given me my first taste (or distaste!) of dementia's emotional roller coaster. One which would soon become an integral part of being mom's caregiver. On the upside, my mother's complete indifference to my taking over her personal business pleased me greatly because it would certainly make my job much easier. All fears of invading her privacy could be permanently put to rest. On the

62

downside though, that same indifference deeply saddened me because it was evidence of the loss of mom's ego – her sense of self. I recognized another piece of her was gone.

My mother participated in our new online banking endeavor only once, during which time she sat quietly by my side, staring blankly at the computer screen. I knew she couldn't comprehend it, but she nodded continually as we reconciled her checking account. Jinx signed her name, Josephine Scribner, on the bottom of each check for the last time on that day. She never again inquired about her bills nor her banking, and I signed all her checks myself.

In order to fully take charge of my mother's money, I needed to become her legal medical and financial agent. I called a longtime friend of mine, who worked for a law firm, and asked her what I needed to do. She offered to bring over a Durable Power of Attorney (POA) form for us to sign and notarize for me.

"Did your mother already appoint you?" my friend asked. "I don't want to drive forty miles to Fountain Hills for nothing."

"My mother is past the point of consent – I appointed myself!" We both laughed.

She had no problem with the arrangement because, as my close friend, she knew none of my siblings wanted the duty, so there would be no legal challenge. The following day, I became mom's POA, with the legal ability to make all decisions regarding my mother's finances, health, and welfare.

Prior to taking over Jinx's money, I had no reason to believe she wasn't paying her monthly bills. I noticed the supply of postage stamps she kept in the kitchen drawer were replenished regularly, and I saw her put four "windowed" envelopes out in the mailbox each month. I also felt *fairly* knowledgeable about her income and savings: Mom received approximately $1,200 each month (Social Security plus an annuity), and she had a CD account which contained about $90,000 from the sale of her house in 1993.

Her other expenditures included about thirty bucks a week spent on specific grocery items only she ate, such as white bread, whole milk, instant coffee and a stockpile of sweets. She also paid me $300 cash, in rent each month.

I know what you're thinking... Yes, I charged my mother rent! When she initially moved in with us, we actually needed the extra money due to Arizona's bleak economic conditions. Jinx's monthly rent and utilities in her own house had totaled more than that, so she was happy to pay us instead. But over the years, even during times when we didn't really need it, I still took the money. The reason stemmed from the deep resentment I harbored since my adolescence – when she made *me* pay *her* rent to live at home, as of age sixteen.

Mom demanded a flat twenty percent of my net paycheck. I'd bring home twenty-five dollars a week from my part-time, after school job and she'd take five bucks of it. With the remainder of my check, I paid all my own living expenses including clothes, gas, and car insurance (imagine money going that far today). Despite my obvious contention that, as a high-school sophomore, I really had no other place to live, she remained steadfast in her ridiculous reasoning.

"Don't you think what I do around here for you is worth five dollars a week?"

To which I logically countered, "I'm your financial responsibility until I'm eighteen!"

Naturally, my argument carried no weight. I had no say in such matters, circa 1976. But twenty years later, as her landlord, I sure did, and I ran with the revenge ball to even the score. Though I'm not proud of it, I have to admit, sometimes I derived satisfaction from thinking, "Payback's a bitch old lady!" Obviously, now, I was going to have to cut her some slack.

Within the first couple days of my financial snooping, I encountered an alarming surprise: The $90,000 I *thought* mom had in a CD account, was in reality only $60,000. The $30,000 difference had become the annuity payment which now supplemented her monthly social security income. I suddenly had a vague recollection of the investment decision my mother made two decades earlier. I'd totally forgotten about it, so it was a shock to learn her monetary assets were a full *one third* less than what I remembered.

This discrepancy gave me greater cause to worry about her financial stability, specifically regarding her long-term care. I had no idea what in-home health professionals or nursing homes cost. She was going to have to pay somebody at some point. Would she be able to afford it when the time came? This prompted my decision to search for ways to shore up my mother's finances. But Jinx was already an extremely frugal woman; I'd even use the term penny-pincher. I didn't have much hope of finding a lot of extraneous expenditures, but once I started combing through mom's boxes full of financial papers, I found plenty.

The first unnecessary expense I discovered was mom's Medicare supplement insurance. The policy made sense when she initially took it out because she owned a home, which needed protection in the event of a catastrophic illness. Now, without a house, it no longer benefited her. As I looked over the yearly payouts from the policy, I could see they averaged little more than one-hundred dollars. Mom's Medicare coverage paid almost 100% of all her health costs. She had no idea she was wasting over two-grand a year on the irrelevant policy. I canceled it immediately.

A cursory glance through my mother's bills revealed she was also needlessly paying my brother Billy's monthly car insurance bill. That became the second item on the chopping block. I called him and told him he had to pay it himself. Done. Well, not *totally* done. The discovery bothered me enough to do some further digging into exactly *how* generous Jinx was being with her money.

Sure enough, I identified a number of sporadic cash withdrawals from mom's bank account occurring on days when I was at work. Mom certainly hadn't driven herself to the bank. I suspected I wasn't the only family member who noticed our mother's new, overly complacent nature. I feared her dementia was turning her into an obvious soft-touch with money and an easy target.

I also unearthed a swollen billfold – containing $1,500 cash – hidden in the back of mom's dresser drawer, under a stack of handkerchiefs. It was a different wallet than the one she carried in her purse. Three weeks later, when I checked it again, more than half the money inside was gone.

Both my brothers had a history of ongoing financial problems. Through the years, mom kept a running tally of the money she lent to them, despite probably having no realistic expectations of being repaid. Occasionally, she prudently turned down their monetary requests with the explanation, "I don't have it to give this month," but now, with her sound judgment and prudence both AWOL, I feared her money might be heading the same way.

Billy and Jaime weren't thieves, and they weren't deliberately trying to hurt their mother, but neither seemed concerned about the looming costs of her long-term care. When she handed them cash, I doubt they thought anything besides, "Mom's okay with it, so she must have enough money."

Jinx had never taught her two sons how to manage money – she did it *for* them well into their twenties – leading them to believe that would be the responsibility of their future wives. My brothers continued relying on our mother's financial help whenever they couldn't make ends meet, creating a

66

codependent relationship which satisfied Jinx's need to be needed. Thirty-plus years later, not much had changed.

I decided to seek answers from our bank for ways to prevent Jinx from withdrawing her own money. To my disappointment, the account manager informed me the only way I could revoke her signing rights was to establish legal guardianship of my mother, which was a far more complicated process than completing a simple POA form and required hiring a lawyer.

Before I could finish expressing my dissatisfaction with that course of action, the resourceful woman offered an alternative solution to me. She suggested I open a "holding account" for Jinx's money – one with only my name on it. Mom's two monthly direct deposits would still go into our joint account, but after the money cleared, I could easily transfer the bulk of it over to the new holding account and pay all of her expenses from it. Thanks to the smart but simple work-around, I escaped the expense of a lawyer during my entire stint as mom's caregiver.

On the account manager's advice, each month I left a scant sum of $25 from mom's income in our joint account, which not only halted any generous "loans" she might be inclined to make, but protected Jinx from the likelihood of being bilked by unscrupulous phone scammers. The holding account also kept my mother's funds from mixing with my own money, which I deemed necessary for propriety sake.

With the new plan in place, and our mother present, I called an impromptu family meeting at my house. Then I dropped the ax, informing my brothers no more money would be forthcoming. While announcing that the "Bank of Mom" was now officially closed, I turned to her and said, "Isn't that right, Ma? We need to keep all your money for *you* now, huh?"

Mom smiled devilishly and gave a resounding, "Yep. I need my money!"

My brothers never expressed any hard feelings toward me, regarding this matter. To their credit, it caused no family discord. I think, once they really thought about it, they understood why – as mom's legal financial guardian – I would have to take such measures.

The final bill I eliminated for my mother was her credit card payment. She had carried an original balance of $1,500 for twenty years, only sending the minimum payment (fifteen dollars), each month. A conservative estimate put her total remittance at over $3,600. I figured she and the card company were *more* than squared. I destroyed the card and never sent them anymore money. I knew the banks had no real recourse to hold mom accountable. What could they do? Lower her credit score? Cancel her card? Garnish her wages?

Ultimately, I considered my plan of action a success. In only a few weeks, I got my mother back on her thyroid medicine, secured her bank account, and successfully alleviated all of her debt. If that involved a little bit of "sticking it to the man," so be it!

NO DIAGNOSIS?

After successfully taking the reins of my mother's finances, I naturally assumed I'd have equal success in my new role as her medical advocate. Jinx's Medicare plan provided ample healthcare coverage. Very little money had come out of her pocket to pay for her past medical expenses, including hip replacement surgery, a hospital stay, an ER visit, and physical therapy in both 2007 and 2008. The following year, when it became painfully obvious my mother was cognitively disabled, I figured her insurance would also cover the cost of in-home care for her. I naïvely thought all I needed to do next was get a dementia diagnosis from her primary care physician and a legion of non-profit, healthcare aides would promptly be dispatched to our house like a squadron of flying fairy godmothers. What's wrong with a little wishful thinking?

Astoundingly, my mother *never* received an official diagnosis of dementia or Alzheimer's. In fact, none of her doctors ever used either term when discussing the decline in her cognitive function or the obvious brain shrinkage, clearly visible on her MRI; not openly in her presence nor privately out in the hall. Instead, they used frustrating euphemisms such as "memory issues" and "forgetfulness." Likewise, nobody recommended any type of medication for her because "memory problems were to be expected for a woman in her eighties." Their professional indifference baffled me. Every doctor's visit had an eerie feeling about it – like an episode of the

Twilight Zone – causing me to suspect medical clones from outer space had taken over the earth.

When I first started posing questions to mom's general practitioner, I knew next to nothing about dementia, but I could definitely recognize she had *some form* of it. Her behavior, such as attempting to read books upside down, went beyond "forgetfulness." However, for almost the entire time as her caregiver, I believed she had Lewy Body Dementia, rather than Alzheimer's – due to her shuffling gait and visual hallucinations.

I later learned that when people with dementia hallucinate it's known as *sundowning*, and of course, it's also a symptom of Alzheimer's disease.

Mom often claimed to see Billy in the backyard, when he was not there. She also observed monkeys in the trees and horses on the patio. We even had an elephant living in our fireplace. Whenever she'd point it out to me, I'd reply, "It must be a baby elephant because our fireplace is small."

Mom would nod in agreement, "Yes, it is a baby elephant."

The strange menagerie didn't scare her, but it confused her a bit. I believe it would have been way more upsetting for her to be told, "You're seeing things, Ma. It's not real." Her son's presence outside disturbed her the most, since she didn't understand why he wouldn't come in and visit. In those instances, I phoned Billy, so she could talk to him, which was enough to pacify her.

According to Healthline and Team Select Home Care websites, *sundowning* is also known as "late day confusion" because for many dementia patients their disorientation and restless agitation gets worse in the late afternoon and evening. Doctors and scientists are not sure what causes it.

Sundowner symptoms aside, the chief reason I didn't think mom had Alzheimer's was because I mistakenly believed people who suffered from it were always difficult, mean, and suspicious. Throughout her illness, my mother maintained a pleasant, easy-going disposition, which I thought precluded her from having it. Not until the final year of her life did I learn the truth, when a hospice director enlightened me.

"Of course Jinx has Alzheimer's," she explained. "Your mother has no short-term memory. If a person can't remember eating lunch 10 minutes ago, they have Alzheimer's! Her behavior isn't mean and difficult because it's not in her nature to be that way."

Wow! Why didn't any of her doctors tell me that? None of them ever spoke frankly about her condition or offered me any form of help in the way of information, advice, or support. During one appointment with mom's long-time physician, when I inquired about eventually needing help with her care, she actually rolled her eyes and scoffed, "Good luck with *that!*" And to my complete disgust, when I asked if we could have a private discussion in the hallway, without mom present, she told me I would need to schedule another appointment and discuss it then. I left the office speechless and outraged.

As far as I was concerned, Jinx needed a new doctor, pronto! As soon as we arrived back home, I started calling other MDs' offices, only to hit another unexpected obstacle; they either weren't accepting any new Medicare patients, or the wait was six months to a year. *Dammit! We were stuck with Dr. Dipshitz!* I vowed to be more assertive with her in future visits. During our next appointment, she agreed to refer mom for neurological testing, upon my request.

The morning of the tests, Billy appeared at my front door with his usual cup of convenience store coffee as we were leaving the house. It was not unusual for my brother to spontaneously "pop in" with his gift of banana bread for mom and visit with her for several hours. I always greatly appreciated the time he spent with her. I invited him to join us and he eagerly accepted, so the three of us piled into my Volkswagen.

On the drive to the medical clinic, I had a fleeting notion of how wonderful it would be if Billy offered to take our mother to the appointment while I stayed home and did *anything* else. The impossible fantasy lasted about two seconds, before reality set in: Our mother wasn't a football to be handed-off to another player on the field. Nobody could be my surrogate. Speaking to medical professionals required a certain level of "insider knowledge" about mom, which only I possessed and could accurately relay. We lived together in the same house, which afforded me exclusive opportunities for observing her behavior. The only person who could answer the doctor's questions was me, and only I knew what needed to be asked on mom's behalf. I was *her* voice, which is precisely what being a medical advocate is all about.

Besides, my siblings also lacked sufficient general health and nutrition knowledge needed for the job. My mother's recovery after hip replacement surgery, a couple of years earlier, is a perfect example.

Jinx had been allowed to rehab at home, rather than at a facility, as long as somebody stayed with her, 24/7. Billy generously volunteered for the job and moved in with us for a month. By the end of the very first week, I couldn't help but notice mom's face had a grayish tinge to it.

Upon interrogating both patient and "nurse," both admitted she had been drinking very little water – despite her daily, toxic intake of post-surgical prescriptions. I suspected our modest mother had purposely curtailed her urination to limit her trips to the toilet with her son, hoping to spare them both the embarrassment.

When I informed my brother of how much she should be drinking, as well as the amount of fruits and vegetables she should be eating for their water content, Billy's reply was priceless.

"Oh, I make sure she gets plenty of fruit. I bought her watermelon Jolly Ranchers, cherry Twizzlers, and Fig Newtons, which have fruit in the middle." He was absolutely serious.

After recovering from my astonishment, I immediately created a required menu for mom and told them they better follow it to the letter, and get over their shyness, otherwise I'd be sending her to the rehab facility. The last thing she needed was kidney failure. There were no arguments, and with only one month of physical therapy, our 80-year-old mother was climbing the stairs without the use of a cane.

Again, such is the role of a medical advocate, but when it came to neurological testing, I was facing uncharted territory.

I had driven past the sprawling, Scottsdale healthcare complex hundreds of times, but never had cause to go inside before. Talk about upscale! With its fine furnishings, chandeliers, artwork, and live, grand piano music, the lobby looked more like a posh hotel than a medical facility. Nobody told us we needed to dress for high tea at Windsor Castle!

I desperately wished I had given more consideration to our appearance before we left the house, but I was trying to get mom ready on time. We may have stood out just a tad! My threadbare jeans and "Uranus Is My Favorite Gas Giant" t-shirt suddenly seemed grossly inappropriate, as did mom's attire: An oversize sweatshirt with giant purple penguins on it, plaid polyester knit slacks, and beaded Indian moccasins.

I normally encouraged her to choose her own outfits – for a sense of personal autonomy – but I regretted not steering her toward something less conspicuous that morning. Moreover, adding to her odd appearance, there was the matter of her arm, which as a result of her refusing to do the required physical therapy last year, had remained bent at the elbow across her chest – as if in an invisible sling.

Then there was Billy, who sported menacing biker gang garb, despite not actually owning a motorcycle. His dyed black, shoulder-length hair was not exactly a common look for a sixtyish man. I got the distinct impression his skull and crossbones bandana, dark glasses, and leather vest may have been a wee bit frightening to some of the senior citizens at the clinic. Suffice it to say, the three of us definitely stood out…but not in a good way. I could almost hear the whispers throughout the hushed corridor, "Oh dear…who let *those* people in here? Perhaps we should call security."

My self-inflicted paranoia and embarrassment prevented me from asking directions of the mannequin-like fashionista at the information desk, imagining her probable snooty response, "Yes, the *freight* elevator is over there…" Instead, we checked the directory and figured out where we needed to go on our own.

We found the *regular* elevator and piled in. On the ride up, the doors parted open onto another floor, where a refined, white-haired, older lady stood waiting. She took a step forward to get in, but then her eyes widened as she surveyed our little threesome – as if she'd encountered the Addams

74

Family. Then she suddenly stepped back out. "I'll catch the next one," she said. The doors closed shut again, my suspicions validated.

We followed the sign to the neurology department and checked mom in for her appointment. An administrator handed her a multi-page questionnaire and told her to fill it out, unaware she was incapable of doing so. Waiting in the multi-rowed seating area, Billy kept our mother amused with jokes about farts and other bodily functions. That was fine with me as long as they kept their giggles and snickers to a minimum, so I could concentrate on completing the forms.

The comprehensive scope of the questionnaire impressed me. It asked for in-depth information on mom's sleep patterns, moods, diet, hygiene habits, and entire medical history. I squeezed in as many details as would fit, in hope of providing a complete picture, and thus, maximum insight into her cognitive function. My optimism began to grow, for the first time; the neurological tests would undoubtedly confirm my mother's dementia and hopefully what type she had.

After about an hour wait, a smiling nurse with a clipboard appeared in front of the waiting area and called out, "Josephine?!" The three of us stood up, and I handed her the completed forms.

"Our mother prefers to be called Jinx," I quickly corrected the nurse.

"She does? Well, hi Jinx! Can you tell me your date of birth?" she said, while escorting us down the hallway.

"December fourth," mom replied.

"Do you know what year you were born, Jinx?"

"No," mom giggled.

"How about 1926?" asked the nurse. "Does that sound right?"

"I guess so," mom laughed again.

The nurse scribbled something down in the paperwork as she led us into a nondescript office. "Please have a seat. Doctor Robards will be in shortly," she said as she closed the door. We sat together, somewhat nervously on the sofa, making idle chit-chat while we waited.

The doctor appeared within a couple of minutes and spoke with us informally before beginning the exam. The statuesque man with graying hair had a commanding presence; a crisp, white, lab coat adding to his air of scientific expertise. His "Neurologist" title *alone* was enough to gain my immediate respect. I estimated he had at least three decades of studying the complexities of the human brain and nervous system under his belt. The field of neurology likely produced very few dumbbells.

Dr. Robards began by asking mom if she knew the date and if she knew where she was. She couldn't recall the date, but she stated she was "at the doctor's in Arizona." Although the questions became a bit more complex as he went on, the entire test was extremely remedial. Nevertheless, it was still too hard for my mother.

When asked to draw a clock face, she did so, but forgot the number eleven. The task of adding two, double-digit numbers left her stumped, staring at the paper. She didn't even attempt it; she simply said, "I don't know this." And when the doctor asked, "Jinx, can you tell me what an *island* is?" mom replied, "It's an island." Despite his many varied prompts, she could not expound on her answer, "It's an island."

My mother's responses didn't surprise me, but they were still very unsettling to observe. Ironically, the most disturbing part of the test session did not come from mom's answers; it came from Dr. Robard's. Incredibly, his theories for her cognitive difficulties did not include dementia.

He suspected sleep apnea as the chief culprit, due to mom's daytime napping and loud snoring, and suggested she undergo a sleep study at a local hospital. I had no qualms with his hypothesis. I agreed sleep apnea was probable and problematic, and it may have even *caused* her dementia, but to me, it was water under the bridge. My mother's snoring had remained at a constant buzz-saw volume – be it day or night – for the entire time she lived with us. We could all hear it through her bedroom door!

If sleep apnea was indeed responsible for her deteriorating mental state, the brain damage had been many years in the making, to the point of being irreversible. Did he honestly believe a few solid nights' rest would restore such advanced cognitive decline? We needed to move forward with a diagnosis and either a course of action, or an admittance of no further action necessary. I presented this argument to the doctor, but my words fell on deaf ears. He scheduled an overnight stay in a hospital to perform a sleep study on mom.

Dr. Robard's other hypothetical cause of what he referred to as "Josephine's mental fog" truly left my own mind confounded. He proposed that since mom had gone several months without taking her thyroid pills, the lapse in medication could have been responsible for her failing memory. I found his backward assumption astoundingly ridiculous, so I slowly and patiently described the sequence of events a *second time* to him.

"Doctor, something caused my mother to abruptly forget all about taking her thyroid pill; a pill she has regularly refilled and faithfully taken every single day for almost *twenty years*. She not only stopped taking it out of the blue, she now thinks a chewable calcium tablet is *that* pill. Don't you see? A lapse in her medication didn't cause her memory loss. Her memory loss caused the lapse in her medication. Mom didn't suddenly stop taking her medicine for no reason and *then* start having memory problems. It's the exact opposite!"

Incredulously, the doctor ignored this argument too, restating again how not taking necessary thyroid medicine could cause a decline in cognitive function. It was like talking to a wall, as we went round and round in a discussion not unlike "which came first, the chicken or the egg?" I understood the reasoning behind the need to rule out other possible causes, but why couldn't this highly-educated man at least acknowledge I had a point? *Was he completely dense or what?* In the end, I at least got him to schedule a second MRI (in addition to the sleep study) for my mother for some current images of her brain.

After the testing, as we headed to the parking garage, my spirits sank to a new low, and my opinion of medical professionals dropped another notch. The verbal fencing match with the neurologist had left me exhausted, annoyed, and suspicious. The "big picture" was coming into focus for me now: If mom's doctors acknowledged the truth and provided a dementia diagnosis, all further testing (paid for by Medicare) would be deemed unnecessary and halted. As cynical and sinister as it sounds, there was considerable money to be made from her illness, especially in light of the current national healthcare landscape. I suspected if she were an *uninsured* woman she would have had an immediate diagnosis; "Sorry. Your mother has Alzheimer's. There's nothing we can do for her."

My brother had remained mostly a silent observer throughout the appointment, but as the three of us climbed back into my car, and I continued to complain about "that idiot Dr. Robards," Billy's comment gave me the only comic relief of the day.

"Yeah, I didn't like that guy either. And his test was stupid too! Hell, *I* couldn't even answer most of those questions."

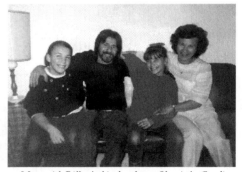

Mom with Billy & his daughters, Sherri & Candi

I NEED HELP!

Despite the many frustrating challenges involved in taking charge of my mother's healthcare and finances, it gave me a sense of pride and empowerment – as if I were somehow taking charge of her disease at the same time. I admit to being a control freak, but it wasn't long before harsh reality set in, thoroughly obliterating my delusions of strength and power and replacing them with crippling anxiety, depression, and fear.

Jinx's mental faculties were declining faster than I anticipated, leaving me with an insufferable feeling of helplessness. I had no idea what to expect next. Distressing scenes of her falling down the stairs, soiling herself, wandering the streets, and dying in her bed occupied my thoughts day and night. I wrestled with serious doubts about my ability to care for her properly, fearing it was way more than I bargained for. *Our lives are going to be turned upside down. What have I gotten my happy little family into?!*

An incurable disease was ravaging my mother's brain and it would continue until her death. The persistent deterioration reminded me of the time I discovered an army of grotesque, giant caterpillars had invaded my garden. There they were, munching away on the underside of almost every leaf, leaving dozens of plants full of holes in their wake. I wasn't able to save my garden, and I wouldn't be able to save my mother either. Contemplating the ongoing, unstoppable devastation of mom's mind was enormously upsetting and emotionally draining. I couldn't bear to get out of bed, dreading each day and feeling guilty for burdening my husband and daughter.

Jinx's rapid decline in short-term memory, not only left me feeling frightened and helpless, it also left me with a young child on my hands. The timing couldn't have been worse. At age fifty, all the splendid symptoms of menopause were now enveloping me. It made me fully appreciate the reason nature ends the childbearing years around the half-century mark: Our patience for children has seriously waned by then! And no question about it, mine definitely had. "Marlene's Bucket List" did not include taking care of a little tyke. I had envisioned my fifties as a wonderful, carefree adventure; full of self-discovery, "me time," and ideally, globe-trotting. Nowhere in the vision was I cutting up my mother's food and checking her adult briefs for wetness.

The mother I knew would have been mortified at the prospect, as well. She always insisted she didn't ever want her children taking care of her. "I don't want my kids wiping my behind! Just stick me in an old-folks home," she would say. But such a thing is easier said than done. If only she had been mean and abusive, it would have been a no-brainer – Goodbye Mommy Dearest!

Jinx was *anything* but mean, however. Mom had the demeanor of a congenial preschooler. How do you put a naïve four-year-old in a memory care facility or nursing home? She wouldn't have been able to understand it. Instead, she would have wondered what she did wrong to make her family leave her alone in a strange, scary place. How terrifying that would have been for her! Ultimately, that's what swayed my decision to keep her; she was more like a daughter to me now. I couldn't abandon her. Making mom leave her home was absolutely out of the question, for the time being anyway.

Luckily, my mother's loyal son-in-law and adoring granddaughter shared my sentiment. It was a unanimous decision, "She took care of us, now it's our turn to take care of her." We all agreed mom would remain in our home, as long as her health and/or safety were not compromised in any way. The Three Musketeers were in it together for the long-haul. We weren't delusional about it either; we realized almost 100% of her care would be on the three of us.

Mom's monthly income and savings could not justify paying for professional in-home care and no help was forthcoming from Medicare. My siblings, who all lived about twenty miles away from us, offered limited participation. They all agreed to "do what they could here and there" to help: Karen could be counted on almost every weekend to take mom to lunch, a movie, and grocery shopping (which she had faithfully done since daddy's passing); Billy dependably kept his regular midweek "date" with mom, arriving early-morning with his gift of banana bread in hand; and Jaime offered much-needed emotional support to me via his daily emails at the end of his work day. He and his wife, Sundie, also stayed at our house with mom for two extended weekends in July of 2011, which was HUGELY helpful. They agreed to relieve us so Harold and I could renew our wedding vows in Las Vegas, with Caitlin in attendance. Even though I appreciated everybody's time and effort, I naturally hoped it would be more.

What I *really* needed, *what my family needed*, were *regular* complete breaks from our never-ending duties throughout the six years before mom went into nursing care. Six years is a long time. Even occasional 24-hour breathers would've been a godsend. What I would have given to hear somebody offer the following:

"Mom can come to my place, for a day or two, so you guys can rest."

81

I wasn't looking for a supreme sacrifice from anybody. But I saw no point in pleading or causing family discord over my siblings' limitations which included car problems, family issues, and their own ill health. I had enough sailing experience to know that when the wind won't cooperate, all you can do is adjust your sails accordingly. The only possible tack then was to lower my own expectations and give up trying to force a higher level of participation.

Perhaps, I should have been flattered. Evidently, my sister and brothers believed me to be the most capable of handling the whole enchilada on my own and trusted me to do so. They were correct in their assessment of my abilities, as well as that of Harold and Caitlin, but the day-to-day, relentless care of our mother, and the mounting responsibilities of the role, were often overwhelming and exhausting. If not for my husband and daughter shouldering the load, I would have had no choice but to place mom in an assisted-living facility right from day one. I unequivocally could not have taken care of her without them – the only two people in the world whose love and dedication to mom, and to me, had *no* limitations.

Despite Caitlin's sincere willingness to help care for her grandma, she (and therefore we) was facing a health crisis of her own: At the age of twenty, and after a year of intermittent, misdiagnosed abdominal pain – which led to a 5-day hospital stay – she was diagnosed with Crohn's Disease. Crohn's is an autoimmune disease which can cause severe inflammation anywhere in the digestive system, and consequently, have a significant impact on a sufferer's quality of life. Essentially, the immune system reacts to food as it would a virus, attacking it with white blood cells. This constant autoimmune response can manifest in an array of problems such as intestinal thickening, poor absorption of nutrients, alternating diarrhea/constipation, mental fog, and extreme fatigue.

Harold and I urged Caitlin to put her health first and sit out the next semester of college to rest and recuperate. She also needed time to mitigate and manage her symptoms, so our sensible daughter smartly agreed it would be best to sideline her education for the time being and remain living at home. But our stubborn little jackass (a term her Grandma Jinx had lovingly bestowed upon her) insisted on maintaining her part-time job as a hair salon receptionist.

Naturally, her condition sent my already high anxiety and worry soaring off the charts. I knew *nothing* about Crohn's Disease. It presented me with another stressful and unpredictable unknown, involving more complicated health decisions, online research, and time-consuming medical appointments. Every eight weeks, Caitlin would need to undergo an intravenous infusion of a drug known to CAUSE lymphoma! It was a treatment with a price tag of $10,000. The insurance complications were a constant nightmare.

I fretted over the monumental task of trying to manage the debilitating illnesses of both my mother AND daughter. Sobbing uncontrollably into my bed pillows upstairs, when Harold and Caitlin weren't home, became a routine part of my day. I always took care to shut the door so my "younger daughter," Jinx, wouldn't hear me either. I didn't want to upset her and make *her* cry too.

Only recently (with the writing of this book), did Caitlin reveal to me how often I cried when she *was* at home. Apparently, I did an abysmal job of hiding my despair, to the point where my own grief-stricken daughter felt compelled to restrain her own tears in my presence – for fear of adding to my already overflowing plate. And worst of all – my seriously sick girl often ended up having to comfort *me* during times she needed my support most. I had no idea. I was on the verge of emotional collapse, as the threads of my mental well-being unraveled into a frayed mess of tangled string.

My precarious emotional state did not override our financial need for me to maintain an income. Two years earlier, my resignation (due to intolerable working conditions) from a full-time, middle school teaching position had serendipitously coincided with the onset of my mother's mental decline. Substitute teaching became the obvious answer for me. The constraints of a standard teaching contract (infinite work hours for abysmal pay) would never allow me the time, flexibility, or energy needed to care for mom, but as a "sub" I had the freedom to choose my assignments and set my daily schedule. Best of all, no after school, long-winded meetings!

Substitute teaching turned out to be the ideal solution for all concerned. I was able to do it the entire time I cared for mom, although the number of days lessened in proportion to mom's cognitive decline. I confess, money was not my sole incentive for working. I needed some normalcy in my life. It's hard to imagine my desperation being *so great* that fighting rush-hour traffic and policing six classes per day – each one filled with thirty-five rowdy teenagers – could possibly be a welcome escape from my caregiver duties. But it was.

Even with taking many precautions to childproof our house, such as removing the stove knobs, we still didn't feel comfortable leaving mom home by herself for too long. After all, it's not entirely practical to keep *every* possible danger out of reach from a 5'3" youngster. How could I possibly have anticipated mom would sharpen her pencil – not with the handy device known as a pencil sharpener – but by whittling it down with a steak knife? These occurrences necessitated the coordination of my substitute teaching assignments with Caitlin's and Billy's schedule: She babysat her grandma on her days off, and he took his shift one or two other days during the week. The bases were pretty well covered.

It's important for me to mention that neither of them *ever* complained about "watching" mom. I know plenty of people whose family members whined or laid guilt trips on them (either outright or passive-aggressively) while helping out, which to me, is anything *but* helpful. I say, if you can't do it unbegrudgingly, shut up, and go the hell home.

The idea of my daughter now babysitting my mother was difficult for me to mentally process. It seemed like only yesterday she was the beneficiary of mom's loving care. The two of them were best buds. As a grandmother, Jinx had much more leisure time and patience than she had while raising her four children. She taught Caitlin how to knit, embroider, and sew; they played hopscotch, drew pictures, jumped rope, and danced the polka. Mom also introduced Caitlin to all her favorite Shirley Temple movies which they would watch together, snuggled on the couch.

Their relationship also thrived due to my mother's radical change in discipline technique. She was not allowed to use corporal punishment or the threat of such on her granddaughter — like she had done with her own kids. Harold and I showed mom it was neither acceptable nor necessary. We parented using our preferred strategy of mutual respect, and my mother had no choice but to follow suit. It paid off for her. There was *nothing* Caitlin wouldn't have done for her grandma.

Despite everybody's help, and as hard as I tried to "keep it together," my emotional dam of despair was at the point of bursting. The festive Christmas season rolled in heavily upon me, serving only to magnify the intense sadness I harbored from watching my mother drift away. I couldn't even begin to face the insurmountable task of shopping for presents (but truthfully, not much was new about *that*). The relentless joy of the holiday turned out to be the final straw, resulting in my complete emotional meltdown.

Poor, unsuspecting Harold returned home from work one particular day, to find me in a bawling heap on the bed, on the verge of hyperventilating into a pillowcase.

"What's going on? Why are you crying?" he said with a genuine look of dismay. He honestly hadn't a clue, but then the male of our species is not exactly known for its intuitiveness. Harold sat down and pulled me close to him, waiting for me to say something, but no words were forthcoming as I continued to weep uncontrollably. I buried my face into his chest, soaking his flannel work shirt with my tears. Finally, all cried out, I sniffled my confession to him.

"This is too unbearable for me. I can't handle watching mom get worse and worse."

Harold tried to comfort me, "What can I do to help you? You know Caitlin and I are here for you (our daughter shielded him from her grief, as well). All you have to do is tell us what you need done. We're in this together, remember?"

"I don't think you can help me. I need *mental* help. I feel like I'm having a nervous breakdown."

"You're not having a breakdown. You're just upset right now." Harold meant well by downplaying my feelings, but it wasn't helping.

"I think I need to go on medication, like an antidepressant, until I can come to grips with this situation."

Harold didn't understand. "Why do you need to take drugs? I thought everything was going pretty well. What happened to make you start crying like this all of a sudden?"

"I cry like this *every day* – that's why I need help!" I could feel my tears begin to well-up again. "You and Caitlin are great, and I know I'm lucky to have you guys, but I feel like my brain is short-circuiting. I'm so emotionally drained. I really need to see a doctor."

86

I felt ashamed of my weakness and for wanting a magic pill to help me endure my life. I knew talking to a therapist would be useless. What could *anybody* possibly say to make me feel better? Nothing would change the situation and the inevitable outcome. But I thought perhaps an antidepressant would provide a mental buffer or cushion to help soften the emotional blows I was experiencing daily. I needed a way to adjust to my "new normal."

Harold never fully comprehended my decision to mentally numb myself, but he supported my choice. I made an appointment to see a nurse practitioner, and during my first session, she gave me a one-month, free trial of the antidepressant Lexipro. Sitting on the cozy sofa of her cheery Scottsdale office, my spirits began to lift somewhat – until she offered this little tidbit:

"The most frustrating thing about dementia is the fact that there's no time-table for its symptoms or duration. You can't predict when the next shoe will drop, what type of shoe it will be, or when the shoes will stop dropping. Since your mother is physically healthy, she could conceivably live with her dementia symptoms for another decade."

Yep, as I had suspected, her words did not make me feel better at all – only relieved I had requested medication. I gulped down a "happy pill" before I even got out to the parking lot.

The NP told me it could take up to two weeks for Lexipro to kick in, but thankfully that was not the case for me. Its effects hit me like a ton of bricks in about a half-hour – and it felt magical alright! My ragged brain suddenly flooded with the incredible warmth of the drug's feel-good chemicals like a delicious infusion of joy!

I raced over to the nearest mall to begin my Christmas shopping and nobody was a merrier elf than I! The crowds and snaking check-out lines didn't even bother me. I happily whistled and bopped along to the repetitive Christmas carols playing in every store. A few shoppers gave me some weird looks when I sang along to Mariah Carey's, *"All I Want for Christmas is You,"* and pointed directly at them, but nobody took offense. I was as spirited as a newly transformed Ebenezer Scrooge and "as giddy as a drunken man!"

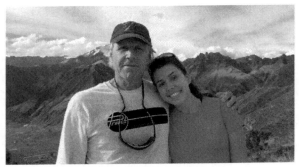

Harold and Caitlin – My Heroes!

PROFOUND LOVE & LOSS

Lexipro helped me coast through the holiday season and usher in the new year without tears. Although it brought me a calm sense of well-being, it also reminded me of the last time I felt the need to deliberately numb my brain with a daily pill: November 24, 1982 – the day before Thanksgiving – the day my father died.

I'll never forget the callous nurse in the hospital elevator. The one who branded her traumatizing words onto my brain forever. "You know, things aren't good up there," she said as she pushed the button for a higher floor. Apparently, she had been assigned to escort us to "Mr. Scribner's room."

"We know." Karen and I choked backed our tears. An hour or so earlier, we had received word via phone call that daddy had gone into cardiac arrest during his angiogram (a test for pinpointing arterial blockages) and had been rushed to the Intensive Care Unit. Billy and Jaime had already intercepted mom and taken her to the hospital with them. My sister and I drove together and fully expected to find the three of them upstairs in the ICU at daddy's bedside.

"Do you know he died?" The nurse stated the question in exactly the same nonchalant tone and manner as one would state the time of day: "Do you know it's ten o'clock?"

Karen and I let out gut-wrenching, plaintive wails as the elevator doors parted open to a corridor, where my mother sat crumpled, weeping into her sons' chests, as they knelt at her side – the three of them in a grief-stricken embrace. Blood ran from a gash in Billy's hand, the result of punching a hole in the hallway wall – his anger expressed on behalf of us all.

My father was not recovering in the ICU. He had not been taken there. It turned out, two of his heart arteries had major blockages, one 90% and the other 95%. Awake during the test, he had watched the angiogram dye course through his circulatory system on the small screen of a monitor. When it reached the obstructions, it sent his heart into cardiac arrest, instantaneously killing him as he lie on the table. I concluded, it must have been hospital policy not to relay such information to family members over the phone, thus the pretense of the ICU story.

My dad's body was laid out in a low-lit viewing room, where we were allowed to visit with him one last time. Everyone else had already done so, except Karen (who didn't want to remember him that way), so I went in alone. While kissing my lifeless father over and over again, my sobbing became so hard and uncontrollable I began hyperventilating to the point of almost fainting. The same unfeeling nurse from the elevator, who stood watch at the back of the room, offered me no kind words or assistance.

I can unequivocally say, speaking for my mother and three siblings as well, it was the most painful day any of us had ever known in our lives. The loss of "my daddy" was inconceivable to me. As a child, he had been my most favorite playmate. Even as a twenty-two-year-old married woman, I still enjoyed spending time alone with him; strumming guitar duets or playing cards. Sometimes I'd even surprise him by hopping on the Phoenix Transit bus he drove, to ride along with him on his route for a few hours.

Upon my father's death, my doctor prescribed me Valium to prevent the stress from worsening my recently diagnosed colitis condition. I had to agree; crying nonstop for hours *does* tend to put a strain on a person's bowels. I numbed myself with the sedative pretty regularly all the way

90

through the following summer. Those months were a complete blur (unlike my Lexipro prescription). I had no choice but to accept an "incomplete" grade in all of my college courses and make them up at a later date. Eventually, somehow, dad's four kids managed to get on with their lives, but his adoring wife, Jinx, would never be the same. She had lost "her Bill" and half of herself along with him.

Although I disapproved of the way my mother limited her world to few people other than her husband, I'm still grateful for the profound gift she inadvertently bestowed upon me. Mom modeled a perfect blueprint for a long and happy marriage. One that I studied, copied, and passed down to my own daughter.

* * * * * * * * *

Jinx Klesik met Bill Scribner at their New Jersey neighborhood hangout, the Manville roller skating rink. They dated for a couple of years and married on Flag Day, June 14th, 1947, when she was twenty and he twenty-two. The newlyweds honeymooned at the Jersey Shore and welcomed their firstborn child, Karen, nine and a half months later. Mom told me the pregnancy happened sooner than they expected because she and daddy were "green horns." When I asked her what that meant she replied, "We didn't know nothin'!"

Their marriage was off to a rocky start. To Jinx's disappointment, she and her new husband had little time alone together. They moved in with Bill's family; his mother, his sister and her husband, plus their 5-year-old daughter.

To make matters worse, Bill liked to go hang out at a local stock car racetrack after work, instead of coming directly home, which did not sit well with his new bride. Jinx's mother-in-law, Molly, butted in often, causing major discord and frequent fights between the young marrieds.

"As long as he earns the money, comes home every night, and doesn't beat you, he can do whatever he wants!" Molly proclaimed, waving her soup ladle in the air. (Yikes! I guess women had lower standards back then!)

Thankfully, not *all* women; not my mother. The final straw for Jinx occurred during a particularly nasty fight when Molly ordered her son to smack his wife "to show her who's boss," and he motioned toward her like he might actually do it.

"That's it. The day you raise your hand to me, I leave!" Jinx yelled.

Then she grabbed her young daughter and left. Mom drove back to Manville, to her parents' house, and asked her mother if she would watch Karen, so she could go back to work. (Go Mom!) The very next day, Bill appeared at the front door pleading with his wife to return, but Jinx had a couple conditions.

"I'll be damned if I'm gonna live with a mama's boy! I'm not coming home with you unless you cut your mother's apron strings. I'm your wife, and you're my husband. You don't take *her* side, you honor *me*."

The second condition was they get a place of their own as soon as possible because she would not be having any more children "under that roof."

Bill apologized and agreed to her terms, and from that day forward both he and Molly treated Jinx with a newfound respect. When the couple eventually bought their first house, Jinx graciously allowed her mother-in-law to move in with them. But before doing so, she told her husband, "Your mother can stay...as long she understands *I'm* the boss of *this* house."

Molly lived with them for ten years, and the two women got along famously. She became the cherished mother-in-law Jinx would later emulate while living with us.

I listened to my mother proudly tell her "final straw" story dozens of times throughout my life. I never tired of hearing it, even though it painted my dad and grandma in a way I'd never personally seen – as complete jerks. I admired my mother for standing up for herself and walking out. Would she *really* have left him for good, or was it merely a bluff? That remains a mystery, but Jinx had a standard for how her husband should treat her, and Bill wasn't cutting the mustard, so she set him straight. All I know is it worked, and her tale of strength and victory had a powerful, far-reaching impact on me – one I carried all the way through to my adulthood.

Between 1954 and 1962, Jinx and Bill celebrated the births of a son, a second daughter (yours truly), and another son. My parents were living the true American Dream. Our eleven-room, split-level house sat on a half-acre lot in the New Jersey suburban neighborhood known as Green Hills. Our huge yard had fruit trees, roses and raspberry bushes, a swing set, and an above-ground swimming pool. Mom stayed home and raised the kids, while daddy supported a family of six on a blue-collar job, with only a sixth-grade education under his belt.

I was keenly aware my dad earned less money than the other fathers in the neighborhood because my parents supplemented his income in other ways to make ends meet. Mom babysat children and did "home perms" for friends. Daddy worked fulltime as a driver for Somerset Bus Company, and did Volkswagen repairs in our garage, as a side gig. They also rented out a bedroom in our home to a border named Bob – a longtime acquaintance of my father's. My parents worked as a team doing whatever they needed to do to support us.

93

My folks were homebodies. They didn't go to cocktail parties or other social functions. Our family piled into the car and went for drives in the countryside on Sundays, usually hitting the park or farmer's market on the way home. Bill and Jinx enjoyed playing with their children, which I think was rare at the time. None of my friends' mothers jumped rope and played hopscotch with them in the driveway. None of my friends' fathers played hide-and-seek with them in the backyard (daddy always cheated though – using our dog, Sandy, to sniff us out).

My father was full of delicious surprises. His job entailed driving a passenger bus from central Jersey into New York's Port Authority Bus Terminal, twice nightly. Every now and then, daddy would drive the bus *home* to take Jaime and me for a thrilling ride into New York City with him (our older siblings weren't interested). I'll never forget the sight and sound of the empty, brightly-lit behemoth bus roaring down our quiet neighborhood street at night, pulling up to the front of our house, right around our bedtime.

He'd plan it in advance with mom, of course. About ten minutes before the prearranged time, Mom would yell at my little brother and me, "Quick, get dressed! Daddy's bringing the bus home!" Jaime and I would squeal with glee as we cast off our pajamas and got back into our clothes. Then we'd go outside and eagerly await our father's arrival on the front porch.

"Here he comes! Here he comes!" we'd shout in unison, hopping up and down.

As we scurried across the lawn toward the loud, conspicuous bus, some of our neighbors would dash out to wave at us from their yards. My brother and I felt like bonafide celebrities climbing the steps to our gigantic coach. Daddy would greet us with a hug and tell us to sit anywhere we wanted. Without fail, we'd run straight for the very back seats, but once his passengers started boarding enroute, we'd always move to the one directly behind his.

Throughout the evening, our dad proudly introduced us to everyone who boarded his bus. "These are my kids – my little girl, Marlene, and my little fella, Jaime." Our favorite part of the trip was driving past The Empire State Building. The following day we'd brag to our friends about how "we got to stay up past midnight."

The fact my dad drove the night shift (from 6pm to 2am) enabled my mother's refusal to maintain her own driver's license. She quit driving when Karen was five years old, which is precisely the same year daddy began working for the bus company. He usually slept until eleven or twelve each day but had a big block of "free time" in the afternoon. Guess who ran all the household errands typically done by a wife back then?

No doubt, most men would have scoffed at such an arrangement, but I never heard daddy complain about it, even when he was obviously exhausted. He could (and would) unapologetically fall asleep anywhere, as soon as he sat down. I recall countless times having to shake him awake from a snooze in the waiting room of my dentist's office, his head collapsed onto his shoulder, drool dribbling down his sweatshirt, and, worst of all, snoring!

Bill had a fascination with cowboys and the Old West. He dreamed of living in Arizona, so he flew out for a weeklong visit – without my mother – to see if we should move there. He fell in love with The Grand Canyon State, and upon his return, my parents put their house on the market. Bill resigned from the Somerset Bus Company after nearly twenty years of service and was given a gold-plated watch for his perfect driving record.

In April of 1973, within days of my thirteenth birthday, we left New Jersey for Phoenix, Arizona. Daddy had no job secured or home for us, but that didn't faze him. More amazingly, it didn't faze Jinx – the ultra-pragmatic woman who had never had a reckless bone in her body. She willingly left behind everything and everyone she had ever known; even her own daughter and new son-in-law. Her reasoning for following her husband's dream was simple, "I go where he goes."

We were all on board for daddy's adventure! It was the first and only trip our family took together on an airplane. The $30,000 my parents pocketed from their house equity felt like a million bucks to them. We stayed in a posh hotel for a full month, with maid service, a luxurious swimming pool, and a doorman. We ate all of our meals in restaurants and spent the evenings at the movies or miniature golfing.

We also searched for a permanent place to live. Home prices were significantly less in Arizona, so my folks could pay cash for our house, with money left over to install a pool. My dad eventually got a job driving a city bus for Phoenix Transit, and mom began babysitting fulltime. Bill worked daytime hours now, but that didn't motivate Jinx to resume driving, so she was stranded at home.

Arizona turned out to be everything my folks hoped it would, but I soon learned of the other reason for our sudden move west: Due to a childhood heart murmur, my dad was certain he would not live to see his golden years. His hairbrained notion had been validated – at the ripe old age of thirty-six – by a gypsy fortune teller at a carnival, who read his palm and predicted, "You will probably not live past fifty...your lifeline is very short." Fearing he would never reach retirement age, Bill decided he needed to find a more peaceful, relaxing place to live; a place where he could "feel like he was already retired." The heavenly beauty of Arizona captured that feeling for him.

96

Sadly, my father's preposterous belief in the fortune teller's words proved prophetic: He died nine years after moving to Arizona, at fifty-eight – never reaching retirement age. Ironically, daddy's physician revealed his heart to be strong, with no trace of a heart murmur. His arteries, on the other hand, were beyond repair from decades of smoking, a diet high in fat, and his sedentary job.

* * * * * * * * *

Most people would agree, if a person lives a life with virtually no heartache for three decades, they are indeed very fortunate. Such is the case for me. The thirty-two years between losing my father and mother were emotionally kind to me. Except for the loss of two beloved canine companions, heartbreak and sorrow had taken a lengthy hiatus. But it had returned with a vengeance, now.

Watching my mom die slowly, a little bit at a time, became as unbearable as that unfathomable day before Thanksgiving, in 1982. Not as inherently shocking, but equally as horrifying – only in a long, drawn-out, excruciating way. Even though my mother's illness afforded me the opportunity to mentally prepare for the end, the final details remained frighteningly unknown. Nobody knew how much suffering she would have to endure or if she would eventually enter a vegetative state.

The difference between my parents' deaths put me to mind of the two ways a Band-Aid can be removed from a wound: My father's had felt like somebody unexpectedly walked up to me and abruptly ripped it off – in one, split-second jerk. My mother's impending demise felt more like someone sitting next to me for months on end...picking at the edges with their fingernails...lifting one tiny piece of the adhesive at a time...with the hairs underneath sticking to it.

97

One way isn't less painful than the other...and they both feel equally cruel.

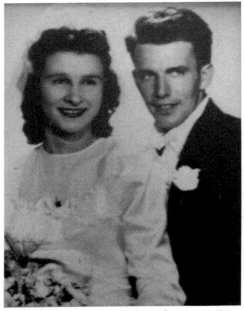

Bill & Jinx's Wedding Portrait – June 14, 1947

COMFORTABLY NUMB
(Beware: A Very Shitty Chapter)

I understand antidepressants are not for everybody. I didn't think they were for me either. Until they were. Lexipro did exactly what I had hoped it would do; it took the edge off an unbearable situation, similar to taking a tranquilizer before getting on a plane.

Even if a person has no fear of flying, air travel is still a nerve-racking experience these days – for the poor sap in economy class anyway. We all have our airline horror stories, and whether it's a Xanax or a couple cocktails, many people require a mind-numbing substance in order to endure it, even if it's only for a few hours.

My stint as mom's caregiver lasted a *bit* longer than a plane ride, but luckily, I only needed to take Lexipro for seven months. In that brief time span, I unexpectedly gained six pounds due to the mindless snacking of cashew nuts and Oreo cookies – something I hadn't done since my pregnancy.

On a positive note, it was that same state of blissful numbness which saved me from experiencing complete mental breakdowns on a daily basis. Lexipro steadied my nerves, serving as much-needed emotional training-wheels to balance me. Over the course of those seven months, it allowed me to *gradually* adjust to my "new normal" and gain the confidence to resume pedaling on my own once again – sans medication.

Developing such a level of unflappability was no small feat. One of the chief reasons for anesthetizing myself, resulted from the terrifying fear of toileting my mother. It was the aspect of her illness I dreaded most, but it was inevitable, and it had finally arrived. Unbeknownst to me at the time, loss of bladder and bowel control meant mom had entered stage six of Alzheimer's, which was *severe decline*. I'd estimate she was three years into the disease at this point.

It was hard to wrap my head around the notion of my mother as a toddler, whom I would essentially be potty-training. Such a concept caused true cognitive dissonance in me. Severe mental discomfort often arises when heartfelt belief conflicts with observable behavior.

I use the word "potty-training" loosely; *training* implies *learning* and mom would not actually be learning anything. Every few hours I would need to ask her if she had "to go potty," and if she said, "Yes," I'd have to take her. If I noticed her already in the bathroom, I'd need to go in and help her. That is *exactly* how you potty-train a toddler. But with mom, there was no anticipated self-sufficiency on the horizon – only increased dependence.

I'd known the role reversal was coming right from the start, but the idea still blew my mind. I would be tending to all her toileting needs, as she had done for me, however, I drew the line at rewarding my mother's bathroom successes with M&M's. Just because she potty-trained her own kids that way, didn't mean I had to!

When it comes to this stage of the disease, my advice can be summarized in one sentence: Brace yourself for the worst and find humor in the horror. I think it's reasonably safe to say the last thing anybody wants to be knowledgeable about with regards to one's parent – with the possible exception of their sexuality – is their private bathroom habits. Anybody faced with this unfathomable task better look for ways to laugh about it if you expect to come away from the situation untraumatized.

This chapter is probably not for anyone with a weak stomach. For those people, I'd probably also have to recommend against caring for a dementia patient *at all* because this stuff comes with the territory. The following examples are not meant to be gratuitous, only to serve as a reality check. This is honestly what a caregiver must be prepared for. It is what it is. You've been forewarned.

* * * * * * * * *

Months before it became necessary, I made mom wear adult, pull-up briefs, as a preemptive strike against her possibly soiling our furniture. I desperately didn't want any messy accidents taking place on our relatively new couch and chair, which were upholstered in soft, orchid-colored leather. Also in anticipation of future trouble – toileting or otherwise – I asked Harold to remove the locks from her bathroom and bedroom doors. I remember feeling so savvy at the time: *I will stay one jump ahead of this disease!* What a laugh! Good try, but unfortunately, I had no idea what I was up against yet.

One day, out of the blue, my mother exited the bathroom carrying her *used* toilet tissue in the open palm of her hand – as if it were a sacred offering to the Goddess of Charmin. She shuffled to the family room and matter-of-factly placed it on the coffee table in front of the couch. Then she sat down and resumed watching cartoons on TV. I was both stunned and sickened in equal proportions. I'm embarrassed to admit my new head-med, Lexipro, was literally *the only thing* that prevented me from screaming, "Oh my God! Are you out of your fucking mind?!" at my poor, demented mother, aka *my little girl.* And NEVER would I have found yelling such a disturbing thing, *at either one*, acceptable. (Perhaps, sometimes at Harold…but certainly not mom!)

Instead, I was able to take a slow, deep breath and approach her calmly, while I tried to assess the best way to address the absurdly horrifying situation before me.

"Mom…it looks like you forgot to flush your paper down the toilet." I said as I pointed at the soiled wad. "That sure is silly. Let's go flush it together now, okay?"

She looked up at me from the couch and nodded, "Yeah, okay." Her innocent smile stung my heart, as always.

Mom grabbed the toilet paper, and I escorted her back to the bathroom where she ceremoniously flushed it down.

"There it goes!" she laughed.

I directed her to wash her hands, and then I sanitized the coffee table with every anti-bacterial cleanser I could dig out from under the kitchen sink. So much for eating dinner in front of the TV on *that* table ever again!

Silly me, I *honestly* believed that was the end of what would later be known among us as "The Toilet Paper Debacle," but it wasn't. It went on for several days in a row. Each time it happened, I went through the same routine with mom: A gentle verbal correction, back into the bathroom, flush the paper, wash her hands, and sanitize the table.

By the end of the week, however, my patience had waned entirely and not only because of the outwardly disgusting nature of my mother's new habit. I had another much deeper concern: The immune suppressant drugs Caitlin was receiving for her Crohn's Disease rendered her at a higher risk for illness. The last thing my daughter needed was to acquire a bacterial infection from a germ-infested coffee table.

To my complete outrage, mom moseyed out of the bathroom once again with her used paper, set it on the table, and nonchalantly plopped down on the couch. *Oh my God! This is ridiculous!* I silently counted to ten, while I seriously contemplated scolding her. In my whole life, I had never verbally disrespected my mother. When I was a kid that was mostly out of fear for my life. But as I stood there now – as the adult in charge – I still didn't want to yell at her. The last thing I wanted to do was hurt her feelings or make her cry. I hated the idea of being mean to my little sweetheart, but she left me no choice – I had to scold her. I couldn't allow this unhealthy behavior to continue. She wasn't the only sweetheart I needed to protect. No antidepressant could offset my anger, yet I was still inclined to treat her with kid-gloves.

"Mom, stop bringing your toilet paper out of the bathroom with you! Please, it's dirty and nasty! It makes me upset. You're going to make Caitlin sick. You don't want to do that, do you?"

She looked up at me from the couch again, this time with an expression of worry, and sadly shook her head, "No."

"C'mon, let's go flush the paper," I said quietly now, offering her my hand.

Back in the bathroom again, she solemnly disposed of it without a word, and foolishly, *once again*, I believed it to be the last time. *Surely, she wouldn't want me to yell at her anymore. She doesn't want to displease me.* Wrong! The next day she did it again, and the one after that too, despite the same stern lecture each time.

Then out of nowhere, the obvious answer came to me. *Duh! I'll make mom a big, bold reminder sign!* My schoolteacher spirit flew into action as I set about creating the perfect bathroom poster. The closet under the staircase housed a treasure trove of Caitlin's art supplies – paint, chalk, colored pencils, and canvases – you name it, she had it. A large piece of blue poster board, magic markers, and a glue stick, plus clipart photos were all I needed for my artistic creation. I attached the finished product to the inside of the bathroom door, so mom would be forced to read it before she came out.

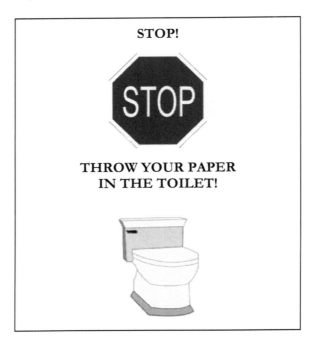

I was proud of my clever poster – it was simple, yet unavoidable. Devising creative ways of motivating mom was always my preference over strong-arming her. I instructed my mother to tell me what the sign said, to make sure she could still read. She did so with ease. Then I reiterated one more time: "What should you *always* do with dirty toilet paper before coming out of the bathroom, Ma?"

Mom answered proudly, "Throw it in the toilet!"

Hugs and high-fives ensued, "Yes! Good job young lady!" Then we linked elbows and moved our celebration to the kitchen for a Popsicle reward party.

While mom and I licked our frozen treats, I entertained a lovely image in my head of President Obama honoring my achievement at a posh White

House ceremonial dinner. "Tonight, ladies and gentlemen, it is my privilege to present the most prestigious and highest award in education to Marlene Jaxon." The POTUS flashes his electric smile as he hands the Oscar-like, gold statue to me. "Ms. Jaxon, you are an extraordinarily brilliant teacher!" I shake his hand and bow graciously to a roomful of applauding A-list celebrities.

The very next morning, my fantasy bubble burst abruptly when mom shuffled out of the bathroom…drum roll please…toilet paper in hand. She placed the gross wad of damp tissue on the coffee table and sat down on the couch. I couldn't believe my eyes! But this time, I said nothing, finally realizing it was pointless to try to reason with her. Nothing I could say or do would alter her behavior. I also concluded she was probably no longer capable of retaining information from one day to the next, so I did the only thing I could: I removed the roll of toilet tissue from the bathroom altogether – along with my "brilliant" new sign. There was no way around it – I would have to clean my mother's backside myself.

During my pre-Lexipro days, an upsetting realization of such proportions would have sent me bawling uncontrollably into my bed pillows. On the medication though, my mental numbness allowed me to take it in stride – as much as possible anyway. Good thing too because "The Toilet Paper Debacle" was only the beginning of our potty plight.

Another major problem that arose, stemmed from my mother's sedentary lifestyle. She and her intestines spent far too many hours folded in half, in a sitting position on the couch. When you don't move, your bowels don't move either. We all tried to engage her in more physical activities, but if Jinx didn't want to do something she stubbornly dug in her heels, shook her head and said, "Nope…I don't want to."

I refused to take "nope" for an answer, so I signed her up for a three-month membership at my gym. I was determined to make her exercise, dadgummit! One of the fitness trainers there designed a sensible work-out that mom and I could do together. My mother seemed to enjoy the new experience initially, but after a few weeks, she refused to do anything other than firmly park her stubborn fanny on the nearest piece of exercise equipment. I couldn't even persuade her to walk on the treadmill for five minutes. The only response I ever got out of her was, "Nope, I'm too tired," so I stopped bringing her. You know the old saying: You can lead a horse to water, but you can't make it do cardio.

Not long after, her lack of exercise resulted in a lower G.I. blockage which required immediate removal at a nearby Urgent-Care facility. Earlier in the evening, I had heard my mother calling my name from her bathroom, prompting me to run full-speed down the stairs to help her.

I threw open the door (no more lock!), "What's going on, Ma?" I needed a moment to catch my breath.

She sheepishly smiled up at me from the toilet, her flannel pajama bottoms scrunched down around her ankles.

"My poop is stuck in my hind-end," she announced with nervous laughter, but thankfully not a drop of shame.

What the hell? Is that even possible? I desperately hoped it wasn't.

"What? Your poop is stuck? Lean forward so I can see what's going on back there..." Pushing down on her back, I took the quickest peek possible.

YIKES, she wasn't kidding! I could see it partially sticking outside of her rectum.

I gently pressed on her belly and instructed her to bear down like she was having a baby. She looked at me like I had two heads. Then I realized why: First of all, she never experienced natural childbirth, having been put under during all four deliveries. Secondly, she no longer recalled the adult

106

events of her life – like getting married or giving birth – and thought of herself as a girl, rather than a woman.

Mom sat there helpless, looking to me for a solution. She couldn't push it out, nor retract it back in. I had only seen such a predicament one other time, and it involved our cocker spaniel and a hunk of steak bone. My mother now resembled the pitiful critter, staring up at me with her big, brown puppy-dog eyes. That incident had also required an expensive emergency removal, *plus* a humiliating lecture from the vet about the dangers of giving bones to dogs.

The doctor at the Urgent-Care gave mom a stool softener to take daily, which I figured would solve the whole sticky problem. No such luck! After a few days of taking it, she had another type of lovely surprise for me.

On that particular morning, in the middle of mindlessly brushing my teeth, an unfathomably foul odor wafted into my nostrils. I froze for a moment, before rinsing and slowly setting my toothbrush down on the sink. I wandered down the hallway, sniffing the air. *What the hell is that putrid smell? Did a packrat die inside our air conditioning vent again?* It seemed to be emanating from down below. When I peered over the staircase, I saw no sign of mom in her usual seat on the couch. I ran full-speed down the stairs (for the second time that week) and followed the rotten odor all the way to her bathroom. Lo and behold, I discovered my mother's stool softener had indeed gotten her bowels moving – all over her *and* the bathroom.

The door was wide open, and she was perched on the toilet again, wearing her usual childlike smile.

"I guess I shit myself," mom giggled. "I made a big mess, huh?"

"Oh my God, Ma," I choked, "you sure did!"

I couldn't believe it. It was all I could do not to cry. I covered my nose and mouth with a washcloth to keep from gagging and surveyed the

107

devastation around me, mentally declaring it a disaster area worthy of FEMA assistance. "Big mess" was a HUGE understatement – *horrific intestinal explosion* would be more like it! I didn't know what to clean first.

Jesus Christ! How could so much crap come out of this little woman? I quickly stripped down my mother, got her safely situated on the shower bench, and turned on the warm water. Handing her the spray nozzle, I showed her how to rinse herself, so she could be doing so while I tossed her unsalvageable, saturated clothes into a heavy-duty garbage bag. No way were those going in my washing machine! I tossed the bag outside the backdoor and quickly opened all the downstairs windows to help rid my house of the overwhelming stench. Then I returned to the scene of the nuclear meltdown to finish mopping up the bathroom and my mother. *Damn those stool softeners! Is this what the doctor meant by "keeping her regular?"*

I decided to shelve the stool softeners, for the time being, opting instead to focus on changing Jinx's diet. Despite foisting fiber-filled meals, fresh fruit, and endless glasses of water upon her, mom began producing stools with the consistency of petrified wood. Little-known fact: Standard toilets can't handle petrified wood. My mother's "deposits" were becoming deeply wedged inside the bowl on a regular basis. The abhorrent task of plunging the nauseating mess was an anxiety-filled ordeal even my faithful Lexipro could not soothe away.

Most of the time, my attempts at un-jamming the blockage were futile, with little to show for my efforts besides a feces-splattered robe. That's when my super-hero husband, Harold, would come to my rescue: Without complaint or fanfare he'd don elbow-length rubber gloves and remove it manually. Yes, *manually*. More often than not, he performed this duty within minutes of coming home from working outside in the brutal summer heat of Arizona. My dear man never *once* made me feel guilty in any way about having to care for my mother. He calmly and matter-of-factly did whatever needed to be done. After all, according to Harold, "That's what you do for family."

Luckily, we did not have to endure this dreadful situation for very long.

I half-jokingly asked my hubby, "Don't they make any supersonic, heavy-duty toilets?" The following day, he burst into the house after work with a huge box balanced on his shoulder (no, he wasn't wearing tights, a mask, or a cape!) and an equally large smile to match.

"I've got something even your mom can't plug up!" he announced.

"Powerful Enough to Flush A Bucket O' Golf Balls!" was the claim printed on every side of the box. Harold installed the toilet in Jinx's bathroom, just in time for her to christen it. As promised, the impressive commode achieved the unimaginable – *WHOOSHING* away the entire contents with unprecedented force and swiftness.

Although the new miracle toilet worked wonders, mom's "stools of stone" were still of serious concern. Through trial and error, I learned altering her diet wasn't enough to mitigate the problem. Additionally, she needed the daily stool softener to keep things moving properly, but its explosive side-effects were prohibitive. We absolutely could not have a fecal time bomb walking around the house. With no easy solution, I was trapped between a rock and a hard place.

Finding an acceptable balance between the two extremes created an internal struggle for me. How much repulsion was I willing to endure (and subject Harold and Caitlin to) in order to keep mom's bowels "regular?" Answer: Not much!

Ultimately, I settled on a somewhat happy medium, giving her the softener only twice a week – rather than every day – because it was easier on my family and me. Sometimes, you have to accept "easier" as the best you can do.

WITH A LITTLE HELP FROM MY FRIENDS

When I say I devised creative ways to motivate mom, I mean I pulled out ALL the stops. Whenever my mother's behavior turned obstinate, I found my most powerful weapon to be humor. Laughter turned her to putty in my hands, so I used everything in my arsenal to crack her up. Nothing was off-limits – bathroom humor, burps, armpit and fart noises, jokes about her droopy derriere – you name it and I did it. I didn't give a rat's ass about political correctness or decorum.

People with Alzheimer's disease live fully in the present, so their lives are a series of moments strung together. I found that to be a sweet, silver-lining to mom's illness, and I took full advantage of it by concocting ways to make those moments as wonderful as possible for her – even if they couldn't be memorable.

My mother's lack of short-term memory also worked in my favor. I could tell her the same joke at every meal, and it would still tickle her funny bone. Even though mom's new playful and easygoing demeanor stemmed from her declining mental function, I thoroughly relished it. The more childlike Jinx became, the more she laughed, especially at the kind of things kids find humorous: Anything gross such as boogers, naughty body parts and doggie doo-doo, and anything goofy or silly. She especially enjoyed physical, slapstick comedy, so I'd purposely pretend to stumble, trip, or drop something (always with overly-exaggerated movements) just for yucks. "Boy you're clumsy!" she'd giggle.

Mom's *adult* characteristics – inhibition, fear, and ego – gradually became replaced with a lovely sense of curiosity, tolerance, and downright silliness. Her once rigid, controlling nature melted into a newly relaxed "whatever" attitude. The proverbial stick had finally been removed from her butt (sorry, Ma!), allowing the spirited and playful Jinx to appear at last!

I liked my new cool mom. The one I'd known my whole life had always demanded the car windows rolled-up because, "The wind messes my hair!" she'd complain. Suddenly, she didn't care. She enjoyed the wind now, joyfully exclaiming, "That tickles!" A freer woman had emerged. On Caitlin's twenty-first birthday, Jinx – the former teetotaler – even drank champagne! I found her new zest for life refreshing and long overdue.

The issues of the past drifted away as we laughed together more raucously than any other time in our relationship. Our differences seemed irrelevant now. The present was all mom had, so I felt driven to make the most of it. That drive fueled my creativity. Who would have guessed I could be such a side-splitting comedian?

My creativity was also derived out of sheer desperation. I needed my "child" to listen to me. I needed her to follow my instructions. What do you do when your grown mother sticks her tongue out at you and ignores your repeated requests for a diaper change? You can't send her to her room for a "time out." You can't take away her TV time. The parenting techniques I'd used on Caitlin were useless.

That's where my "friends" came in; the colorful cast of characters I invented to help coerce my mother into cooperating with me. Since she got the biggest kick out of exaggerated foreign accents, the personalities I created were theatrical, ethnic stereotypes (trés un-PC!): Lotus Flower, the Asian salon lady, assisted with personal grooming; Maggie, the English Lady in Waiting, was her bathroom and wardrobe attendant; Francois, the romantic Frenchman, escorted her to dinner; and Luigi, the Italian pizza maker, helped with diapering. Their performances were basically the same each day, but it was all new to mom, so she laughed every time. I got a lot of mileage out of the same comedic routines.

I created the character of Lotus Flower while attempting to trim my mother's gnarly fingernails. She had always worn her nails long and probably thought they still looked glamorous, except now they were thick, jagged, and discolored. Keeping them well-manicured became a huge challenge for me because she'd stubbornly jerk her hand away every time I applied the nail-clippers to them. My repeated pleas were met with defiance. Folding her arms tightly across her chest, she'd shake her head and say, "No way." That pissed me off to no end, but what was I to do? Pin her down and forcibly manicure her? I quickly dismissed that idea.

Humor saved the day, once again, as the solution came to me in the form of Lotus Flower.

"Oh pretty lady, you gimme hand, and I make beautiful nails for you."

Lotus Flower's lilting voice and gentle ways were enough to distract mom. She became so spellbound by her, she'd relax and willingly extend her hand. Jinx especially enjoyed the soothing, fragrant hand massages.

"Here, let Lotus Flower rub some nice lotion on you, sweet lady. Your skin is so soft and young – like baby bottom." It worked like a charm every time.

English lady-in-waiting, Maggie, not only cleaned and dressed mom but also gave her the royal treatment throughout the day. Naturally, my mother basked in the praise and adoration Maggie bestowed upon her.

"Oh goodness mum! Don't you look lovely in that new sweater? Let's go show it off around the palace, shall we Princess Jinx? C'mon love!"

Then mom would take my arm and assume a stately posture as she paraded through the house with Maggie. Smiling and waving, she greeted her royal subjects around the castle, "Hello, people!"

Literally overnight, my mother went from coming to the dinner table when called, to remaining on the couch in confusion. Her "deer in the headlights" look told me she wasn't trying to be difficult or obstinate. She was struggling to process the meaning of my words, but they weren't sinking in. Rather than yelling, "Dammit, Mom! Are you coming or not?" I conjured up the always-charming Francois to help me. And I have to say, she appeared to understand *his* words just fine – even with his accent. My father may have been her number one boyfriend, but she sure did enjoy the romantic attention from her dreamy Frenchman.

"Ah ma Cherie, you are looking most enchanting zees evening." Gazing deeply into her eyes, he would take her hand in his and pepper it with kisses, up her arm and all the way to the elbow – ala Pepé Le Pew, the romantic *Looney Tunes* skunk. "We shall run away togezer, eh my leetle cheeken? But first, will you do me zee honor of joining me for dinner se soir, ma petite dumpling?"

Then Francois would help mom to her feet, and slowly waltz her over to the kitchen table while humming softly into her ear. In a final gallant gesture, he'd pull out her chair for her and make sure she was comfortably seated before sliding it back in.

"Bon appétit Madame." Francois would blow her a kiss before bowing out of the room. That sexy guy *definitely* had a way with women.

Luigi made his appearance mostly at bedtime, when mom usually resisted the final diapering of the day. She insisted my dad slept next to her each night, so perhaps she was embarrassed in front of "her fella."

Stubbornly planting her butt firmly on the edge of the bed, she'd stiffen her body and refuse to budge. I didn't want to ruin her lovely notion of daddy's presence by arguing with her.

It served no purpose telling Jinx her husband died years ago. How could she possibly comprehend such a thing? That's where Luigi came in. Distracting her with Luigi's antics was way more effective and certainly more fun.

Wearing an adult diaper atop his head as a chef's toque, Luigi would toss imaginary pizza dough high into the air exclaiming, "Mama Mia! I will-a make a pizza for you, Jinx! But only iff-a you put on-a the clean-a pants-a? Yes? And iff-a you say no, then I will-a put-a stinky fish on-a you pizza!"

My mother's lifelong aversion to fish prompted her to quickly surrender to my diapering directions. Each night was pretty much the same act, but it yielded instant giggles and cooperation. And if Luigi happened to throw in a fake fart at the end – even better!

THE $200 BURGER

At least once a month, I'd take my mother to the neighborhood McDonald's. We'd bring the dogs along for the ride and order from the drive-thru. Mom liked to watch the Disney Channel while she ate, so we brought the food home with us. Even though I'm not a fan of fast food, I saw no reason not to treat her to something she always enjoyed – a cheeseburger, fries, and an orange drink. But as Mom's mentality became increasingly childlike, her McDonald's order changed slightly; she now wanted a cheeseburger *Happy Meal* – so she could get a new toy.

Back home, on the couch in the family room, mom would set the red and yellow box on the coffee table in front of her and eagerly dig through the food like a burrowing mole, until she found the prize. Over the years, I had heard my mother describe the Happy Meal toy as "a cheap piece of crap." Now, her youthful eyes saw it as a rare treasure. And it didn't matter what it was – a tiny race car, a Ninja-Turtle, or a mini Slinky – it captivated her to no end.

Mom's scattering of toys around the house took a little getting used to at first, especially since Caitlin's childhood playthings were confined to her bedroom. Over time, however, the miniature space aliens on the coffee table, the stuffed animals arranged on the couch, and the jars of Play-Doh on the kitchen counter became a natural part of our home décor. I confess to spoiling "my little girl" with sticker/coloring books from the grocery store each week – like I did as a young mother.

Mom especially loved the paper dolls I bought for her. She used to draw the clothes for Karen's and my cut-outs, and many years later, for Caitlin's. Jinx had entertained the notion of being a fashion designer when she was a teenage girl, but never pursued it. She retained her artistic ability and drawing talent well into her dementia and still delighted in doing all types of art projects like finger painting and colored chalk designs.

Making a mess, in pursuit of creative activities with mom, was never a problem or even a consideration for me. But my own carefree attitude on the subject often triggered some childhood resentment, remembering how my mother's compulsion for an ultra-clean house stifled *my* creativity and fun.

Jinx had extremely rigid rules. With the exception of crayons and colored pencils, the use of art supplies was taboo in the house. A spotless, uncluttered home was paramount. Most days, my little friends weren't welcome inside. Occasionally, she allowed me to bring *one* of them in, but we could never play up in my bedroom. Mom didn't want them "traipsing around everywhere," so they were relegated to the downstairs playroom. This was only one room further into the house than our family dog was allowed to go. And if any of the little moochers requested a drink (even water) or a snack, they were SOL. Mom directed me to tell them to go home and get one. "I'm not feeding the whole damn neighborhood!" she'd usually proclaim within earshot of them. Needless to say, inviting any kids for sleepovers and birthday parties was out of the question.

It was difficult trying to keep those memories at bay, while remaining "in the moment" with mom. It took a conscious and concentrated effort to ward off my latent bitterness. *Let it go already, Marlene!* Lucky for mom I wasn't a vengeful person, or I might have made her eat in the kitchen, instead of letting her enjoy her Happy Meal while watching *Hannah Montana*.

One day, while she happened to be doing exactly that, I decided I'd let her watch her show while I watched *Judge Judy* in my bedroom. Mom and I used to watch *Judge Judy* together each day after I got home from work. She'd always tell me how the blunt judge's snide remarks sounded like me and loved it when Judy rudely yelled at the litigants.

"What is the nature of your disability, sir? A bad back? Obviously not bad enough to keep you from making six children! Maybe you should find a new hobby!"

Mom would laugh and tell me, "That's something you would say!"

I still miss those times, and I regret taking them for granted. My mother's interest in the real-life court cases waned once she started losing her ability to understand reality television programs and adult situations in general.

Upstairs in my room, Truman, my little Maltese-mix pup, joined me on the bed in front of the TV. Suddenly, and for no apparent reason, he began wildly running around, panting, and shaking. He climbed the pile of pillows at the headboard and clawed at the wall, as if trying to escape an invisible predator. His giant pupils dilated with intense fear, his pink tongue leaving a saliva trail on my comforter. The poor guy seemed terrified, almost to the point of hysteria.

I had only seen Truman behave this way once before, when the ceiling smoke alarm started screeching in the middle of the night. I had to sit with him and our mini-schnauzer, Roxanne, out on the balcony, while Harold frantically retrieved a ladder and a new battery. The high-pitched noise had caused both dogs to go ballistic.

This time, our smoke alarms were silent and so was Roxanne. Even more strange, about two minutes later, Truman was perfectly calm again, curled up at the foot of the bed. I couldn't imagine what might have spooked him. Maybe, like Harold, he simply couldn't stand Judge Judy's caustic criticism?

About a half-hour later, it happened again. This time he sprang from the bed and headed for the balcony door. He continued trembling and panting uncontrollably while I cradled him in my arms. *What in the world is causing him to freak out?* A few minutes later, he acted as though nothing had happened.

His behavior reminded me of the epileptic fits our cocker spaniel, Chauncey (the dog with the bone stuck in his arse), used to have. His seizures and Truman's panic attacks were almost identical. I called our veterinarian, who recommended I bring him in immediately for bloodwork, which I promptly did. Roxanne went along for support, but I left mom home since the office was only two-minutes away. Truman displayed no signs of distress while at the vet's (other than his usual shaking like a leaf).

When we returned home, Harold was exiting his work truck and asked me where I'd been. As the dogs bounded out of the backseat to greet him, I relayed the details of Truman's episode, the vet exam, and the possibility of our little guy having epilepsy.

"Great...and how much did that hairy, little beast cost us now?" Harold joked, as he kissed me hello.

"Two hundred dollars," I cringed as I said it. "Truman seems okay at the moment."

Harold scoffed again, "Well, he better have *something* wrong with him for *that* much money!"

We went inside and headed downstairs with the pups following closely behind us. Mom was still seated on the couch, right where I'd left her; watching the Disney Channel, with the remnants of her Happy Meal in front of her. She seemed oblivious to the fact I had left and returned. Harold thoughtfully stopped to chat with mom about her day, as I led the dogs through the house to feed them dinner. From the kitchen, I could see

119

my mother was showing Harold her latest McDonald's toy, but I couldn't quite make out what it was.

Until I heard it. A very soft, but shrill, RING-RING. A few moments later, another RING-RING. Mom's new toy was a plastic customer service bell! Mom batted it quickly, two more times, with the palm of her hand and giggled – RING-RING. Although high-pitched, the bell wasn't loud, since it wasn't metal. The sharp, piercing chirp sounded similar to that of a cheap, plastic whistle. And then it dawned on me…similar to a dog whistle; the kind *only dogs* could hear. Somehow, Truman was able to hear the high-pitched chirp all the way upstairs, when I couldn't.

Truman instantly went berserk! The terrified pooch raced wildly around the dining room table, whimpering with his tail between his legs before tearing outside through the doggie-door flap. I looked out the window to see him shaking and cowering in the corner of the dog run. Meanwhile, Roxanne (inexplicably unphased by the noise), patiently awaited her dinner.

I ran to the family room to confirm what had just happened. Harold picked up the harmless-looking bell from the coffee table and stared at it in disbelief before taunting me with the obvious.

"So, let me get this straight…Jinx's Happy Meal cost us $200?"

Mom laughed and exclaimed, "Whoa! Boy, that's *some* hamburger!"

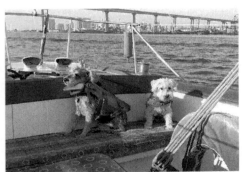

Roxanne and Truman – sailing in San Diego

MY LIFEBOAT

Do you *really* need to take Lexipro anymore?" I asked myself, as I popped the pill into my mouth. I swallowed it before deciding, "No, you don't."

After seven months of taking the antidepressant, I easily – but gradually – weaned myself off it over a span of three weeks. The drug had served its purpose, providing me a comfortable mental cushion for adjusting to my often unbearable caregiver duties, and the unpredictable timetable of mom's disease. The prescription also helped me with what counselors call *anticipatory grief*, the sadness caused by witnessing uncertain, day-to-day loss of a loved one. By the end of summer, I felt a new sense of resolve about my ability to face mom's illness head-on, without daily medication.

Within a couple of months, however, I realized I still had a desperate need of some type of relief but preferably something other than pharmaceutical. I longed for a place where I could get away from my relentless responsibilities. A tropical vacation sounded like the ideal retreat, so I sent my heartfelt wish out to the cosmos and visualized myself on a South Pacific island every chance I got. In a few short weeks, the universe answered me – in the form of a sailboat.

Harold's sister and her husband owned three older boats, which were docked at a harbor in downtown San Diego. The three pricey, marina slips had become burdensome to them, as had the perpetual nautical upkeep.

When they offered to *give* us one of the sailboats, I couldn't believe our luck. Although an avid sailor, Harold didn't exactly share my enthusiasm.

"How can you refuse the gift of a sailboat?" I pleaded.

"Very easily," he laughed. "We can't afford a 'free' sailboat."

My hubby contended that the monthly slip fees, plus the regular maintenance of a 40-year-old, *wooden* sailboat would be way too costly. This prompted me to phone his sister to ask if she'd retain half ownership and expense. She happily agreed, so Harold, realizing he was outnumbered, reluctantly approved the deal. The 41-foot, 1967 Kettenburg sailboat was officially half ours! Woohoo!

The Cantina (we kept its original name) was far from luxurious. It had no air conditioning or heat. There was a two-person sleeping berth in the bow, a tiny galley, a dining salon, and a sliver of a bathroom. There was no shower and no hot running water. The boat's two sinks operated via foot pumps, and the "refrigerator" was actually a wooden icebox. I didn't care. It would be my island paradise.

I started escaping to my sailboat sanctuary about every six to eight weeks. Far more therapeutic than Lexipro, the Cantina became my literal lifeboat – tethered on the bay a mere 380 miles away. Whenever the emotional pressure began to overwhelm me, all I had to do was clear the intended weekend with my compassionate husband and daughter. Once they gave me the green light, I'd pack up my VW and head for the coast.

I didn't have the sailing expertise to sail the boat without Harold, but I didn't need to go asea to relax on it. It may have sorely lacked posh amenities (or basic amenities!) but to me it was the Ritz. Sometimes I invited an adventurous friend along for a "girls' getaway," but most of the time, I went by myself – to satisfy my desire for solitude.

The exhilaration I felt each time I drove into the marina parking lot never waned. No matter how exhausted I was from my long desert journey, catching that first glimpse of the glistening San Diego Bay never failed to energize my soul. Within seconds of arriving, I'd scurry out of my car onto the bay front sidewalk, impatient to feel the cool coastal breezes tousle my hair and invigorate my skin. The graceful, blue curve of the stunning Coronado Bridge spanning the water had a way of coaxing every drop of stress and anxiety from my body.

After a few minutes spent drinking in the beauty of the horizon, I'd snag a marina dock cart (similar to a wheelbarrow) and pile it high with my weekend provisions. Then I'd eagerly make my way down the dock, through the security gates, lugging my heaping load behind me. The hypnotic tinkling sound of metal halyard lines, brushing against their masts, summoned me to where the Cantina sat moored – like a faithful horse awaiting its rider at a hitching post.

I couldn't wait to hop onto my old friend once again and throw open all the doors, hatches and windows, allowing a rush of ocean air to flow through. After hauling my belongings down below, I'd pour myself a glass of wine and sink into the cozy seat cushions of the open cockpit. Aaaaah...just what I needed.

The sight of the late afternoon sun melting on the waves calmed my frazzled nerves and quieted my perpetually overwrought brain. For four worry-free days, I wouldn't have to take care of anybody but myself. The only decision I had to make was what I wanted to eat for dinner: Thai, Chinese, or Italian.

I rarely ever ate in any of the Historic Gaslamp Quarter's wonderful eateries though, – all an easy walk from the marina. I usually ordered my food "to go," preferring to dine on the boat, under the evening stars, instead. During the summer months I even had a free dinner show, as the San Diego Symphony's dramatic orchestrations drifted over from an adjacent park amphitheater, culminating in a spectacular bayside fireworks display.

At night, I basked in the soundest of sleep; the gentle lapping of waves against the hull produced a rhythmic rocking, similar to a baby's cradle. The seagulls' morning squawks were my alarm clock signaling sunrise on the West Coast. Breakfast on the boat provided a meditative start to each day: French press coffee, fresh fruit, and warm oatmeal – enjoyed al fresco from my exclusive waterfront café.

The glorious weather and panoramic scenery provided so many blissful opportunities for renewal of the mind, body and spirit. Some days I'd catch a water taxi over to Coronado Island for some shopping, others I'd spend bicycling the miles of picturesque pathways with the bay breeze in my face. And on the laziest of days, I'd unwind beside the lagoon pool of the marina's parent hotel. Relaxing on a chaise-lounge in the shade of a palm tree, with a fruity cocktail and a great beach novel, was the perfect way to spend the afternoon.

My San Diego visits were always best when Harold joined me, and the two of us could actually enjoy the Cantina in what it was built for – sailing! With him in the role of capable captain and I as his bumbling first mate, we made a comical team (his Skipper to my Gilligan), but we always had a grand time cruising the bay, and whale-watching out on the ocean blue.

Ironically, the heavenly peace I felt while in California always brought with it a bit of internal turmoil, due to my gnawing desire to move back there again. I was an ocean child at heart, and when the sea holds the heart captive, it physically aches to leave it. Living in Arizona made me feel like a fish out of water – gasping for air, in the stifling, hot Sonoran Desert.

Whenever Harold and I went away alone for a sailing adventure, it always made me think about my parents and how they literally *never* took *any* trips without their children. Their vacations consisted of amusement parks, and one day (yes, only one day – singular!) per year at the Jersey shore. A day at the beach was a major expense for them because it included food, rides, and games on the boardwalk. It was *always* about the kids.

Thankfully, for their 35th wedding anniversary, they *finally* went away *alone* together. June of 1982, the four of "us kids" gifted them a weekend getaway to Sedona and the Grand Canyon. Bill and Jinx hadn't taken a vacation, just the two of them, since their honeymoon. That anniversary gift turned out to be of greater significance than we could have ever imagined. Five months later we lost daddy.

Unlike my folks, Harold and I have taken plenty of vacations without our daughter. We never had the slightest concern about leaving Caitlin with Jinx when she was little. Almost two decades later, with Caitlin in the role of baby-sitter, we still had no qualms about leaving her home with her grandmother, while we escaped for a weekend alone.

Her maturity defied her youth. How many college kids would encourage their parents to vacation in San Diego ("You guys should go sailing!") while they babysat their mentally-ill grandmother for four days? Even more rare, how many could handle the responsibility with such a remarkable level of finesse and confidence, that their parents wouldn't be the least bit nervous about leaving? I would wager not many, but ours did.

Clever Caitlin had devised the perfect method for keeping her granny in line, while we were in California. Whenever Jinx defied a request, such as, "It's time for your bath now, Grandma," all our resourceful daughter had to say was, "If you don't listen to me, I'm going to call mom, and then you'll *really* be in trouble." Caitlin never actually needed to phone me. The threat alone was enough to spur her granny's immediate beeline toward the bathroom.

AN *UNAPOLOGETIC* BALANCING ACT

"If you are traveling with a small child or someone needing assistance, secure your oxygen mask first and then assist the other person."

Most people have heard that announcement aboard an aircraft so many times, they no longer listen to or watch the safety demonstration prior to take-off. They understand the obvious logic behind it; you can't take care of the individual in need if you are lifeless. Duh! Then doesn't it stand to reason, that what's true at 35,000 feet is also true on the ground?

Curiously, this commonsense approach never occurs to many caregivers. It may be they are perfectionists who set the bar impossibly high for themselves, or perhaps they're nurturers who thrive on self-sacrifice. In either case, exhaustion and failure are often the end result. As a pragmatic realist, it's almost impossible for me to relate to either mindset, which I wholeheartedly believe contributed to the success I had in taking care of my mother.

Not that I'm devoid of emotion or incapable of making decisions based on gut instinct. I just happen to know ignoring your own needs while providing care to someone else is not a viable plan. Burnout is inevitable – oftentimes requiring medical attention for the *caregiver*. What happens to their vulnerable loved one then? The person most dependent on them? I shudder to think of the repercussions. I remember reading somewhere – perhaps in a fortune cookie or horoscope – the following words of wisdom:

126

"Start with you. If you're not compassionate and kindhearted toward yourself, you'll resent whatever generosity you give others."

I believe that should be every caregiver's creed. I practiced it daily.

The most selfless thing you can do for the person relying on you for care, is to maintain your own health, happiness, and practical life balance. This is *way* easier said than done, of course. Everybody knows caring for a loved one with dementia is grueling – requiring an almost super-human amount of mental, physical, and emotional energy. It's not a job for weaklings. Unfortunately, we have a tendency to judge ourselves too harshly. We're not actually super-human – we can't do it all perfectly.

It's nearly impossible to anticipate and correctly assess the ever-changing needs and abilities of an individual with dementia but take comfort in knowing that even though mistakes are a given, most are not life-threatening. And if any relative has the audacity to imply a lack of diligence or dereliction in duties on your part, there is a simple, well-mannered reply (not involving the middle finger):

"If you think you can do better – be my guest. When would you like to take over?"

Be sure to deliver the question with a smug tone for maximum effect.

On the subject of unforeseen, caregiver mistakes, the following incident comes to mind:

One day, I served mom lunch at the kitchen table, like usual. I felt confident I could easily make a quick run to the bank while she ate her sandwich, figuring I'd find her back on the couch, watching TV upon my return. Wrong! When I got home about thirty minutes later, I discovered mom hadn't moved. Despite having finished her lunch, she was still sitting in the kitchen, staring blankly at the wall, her empty plate on the table in front of her.

"Ma, are you done eating?" I asked.

"Yep," she nodded at the wall.

"Do you want more food?"

"No," she shook her head. "I'm full."

"Why are you still sitting there? Are you okay?"

"I don't know."

"Can you get up?"

"No. The chair is stuck," she spoke as though she were in a trance.

What? She can't scoot her chair back from the table anymore? I stood there for a second, trying to process that new revelation. It was clear mom had turned another corner. Initially, I battered myself with a barrage of guilt and shame for my negligence. *Now look what you've done! The bank couldn't wait till later?*

I punished myself with exaggerated visions of my mother sobbing as she struggled to extract herself from the kitchen table and vowed to be more conscientious in the future. Until I came to my senses, that is, and realized the near impossibility of anticipating mom's sudden inability to perform the simple task of pushing her chair back and standing up. I mentally added it to the already long list of things I had failed to properly predict my mother would do, like eating fake fruit, climbing an unlit staircase in the middle of the night, using a spatula to unchain the front door and escape, and sharpening a pencil with a steak knife, to name just a few. Certainly, any of those things could have had disastrous results. But none of them did.

My advice is to try to go with the flow. Find the humor in it, if you can. Take steps to minimize frustration and anger. Having a realistic, nonreactive caregiving style helped me maintain my sanity. I kept mom's daily agenda small and my expectations reasonable. Tasks were always more enjoyable if I did them *with* mom instead of *for* her or *to* her. And if a snag arose in our routine, so what? It wasn't the end of the world; nobody was to blame. We moved on to something else. There's no sense sniping at a sick person.

128

I have no formal training in elder care. Most people don't. We only have *on-the-job* training! So even if my best judgement wasn't always correct, I found comfort in knowing my dedicated effort enabled mom to remain at home with her loved ones. At the end of the day, I gave myself a reassuring, mental pat on the back and concentrated on resting up for the crazy *new* challenges the next one would surely bring.

Finding the proper balance in caring for mom, my husband, daughter, and myself was an enormous challenge. Spreading ourselves too thin and putting our own needs last is undoubtedly a struggle most women can relate to. The following things helped *me* take care of *me*:

- Maintaining healthy eating habits. I never skipped meals and didn't turn fast food into a regular part of my family's diet. Did we bring home an occasional pizza or bucket of chicken? As mom would say, "You betcha!"

- Exercising regularly. It's a natural mood and energy booster! If I couldn't get to the gym, I put on a favorite CD, and hula-hooped in my kitchen. Sometimes I popped in an old aerobic tape, *Latin Dance Moves,* and cha-chaed around the living room. Mom loved moving to music with me too. She and I also walked the dogs together until her shuffling gait became too prohibitive.

- Social connections. My friendships took on greater importance. It's easy to become withdrawn and isolated, so it's essential to spend time with understanding and supportive people. Don't be embarrassed to ask for help or too ashamed to accept help when it's offered. Feel free to speak frankly about your situation. When somebody asks how you're doing, don't simply say, "I'm fine." Talking is therapeutic.

- Using over-the-counter sleep aids, such as Melatonin, when necessary. I felt no guilt when it came to giving mom a sleeping pill. Allowing her to roam the house at night – like the ghost of a lost soul – risking injury, was not an option. Nor was it acceptable for Harold and Caitlin to lose sleep due to mom's midnight shenanigans. I put an immediate end to it the one and only time I awoke to find her hovering at my bedside like a spooky apparition!

- Maintaining hobbies such as the piano, guitar, and even sailing. When mom took a nap or watched a TV show, I took advantage of "Me Time." Sometimes that simply meant escaping into the pages of a mystery novel – the housework be damned!

- Escapes and breaks. Regular and planned respite is critical for any family. Harold, Caitlin, and I had almost no opportunities for the three of us to vacation together, so we took mini-vacays any way we could. Sometimes Harold held down the fort while Caitlin and I left town; other times, I stayed home while the two of them took off; and once in a while Caitlin watched her grandma while Harold and I got away. I also made a point of regularly leaving by myself for a weekend (see My Lifeboat chapter) – completely guilt-free. I realize not everyone has that luxury or level of support, but I did, so I took full advantage of it with no apologies! *

> *** Side Note:** I'm not out of touch with reality; I understand most people do not have a sailboat as a retreat. However, if I hadn't had the Cantina, I would have found something else; perhaps a short "stay-cation" at a local hotel or a relaxing spa treatment. During times when those type of luxuries weren't feasible, a meditative hike in the surrounding Sonoran Desert served me well. The majestic mountains and welcoming wildflowers soothed my soul and cost me nothing.*

- Lowering my expectations; from ideal...down to pretty good. Some things are beyond our control. We weren't nurses or social workers. We were Jinx's family. We loved her, and we cared for her the best we could. Period.

- Incorporating fun activities, for us to do together, into each day. In other words, playing with her. Playtime was beneficial to us both. Taking a break from the adult world helps keep you young at heart.

- Gathering information from all possible sources, including professional organizations. Educate yourself. Ignorance is *not* bliss. (See resources pages provided in the back of the book.)

- Seeking (and receiving) hospice support even when mom wasn't technically at "end of life." ("The Bittersweet Summer" chapter is devoted to this subject.)

- Making a conscious effort to avoid running on caffeine and partaking in too much "wine time." I must confess, I was not always successful with this one!

- Yoga, meditation and journaling. *

> ** I added this to the end of the list and qualified it with an asterisk because I did not actually do these. In hindsight, I believe they would have been valuable relaxation tools. I deeply regret not keeping a journal. A written account of mom's final years, as they were happening, would've been a wonderful treasure.*

Providing care to my mother also had one unwavering condition attached to it: Compromising my family's finances was a deal-breaker. The Jackson family was not going to wind up in the *poor farm* (old fart terminology) on her behalf. Harold's construction business had taken a hard hit from the 2008 recession. We were still struggling from it and in no financial position for me to be Jinx's 24/7, unpaid nurse.

When I initially committed to her full-time care, I also worked full-time, but I did *not* have discretionary income to throw around. Coming to grips with mom's deteriorating mental state unraveled my own, therefore, as her Power of Attorney, I saw no problem treating myself to a well-deserved, stress-relieving massage on my mother's dime, every few months. As her needs became more daunting, resulting in my near nervous-breakdown, I also used her funds for my monthly anti-depressant prescription and therapist co-payments. Mom's income paid for anything directly and indirectly attributed to her care. I saw no reason why my family's sacrifice should unnecessarily include money.

Over time, as my mother's all-consuming illness necessitated a reduction in my job hours, I proportionally supplemented my waning income with a weekly salary from Jinx's account. I figured she had two choices – pay me or pay a nursing home. Nobody wanted the latter for her.

I had informed my siblings I still *needed* to work, and if none of them could care for mom Monday through Friday to enable me to do so, then the money in her savings (from the sale of her home) would gradually get consumed in the form of my own compensation for the full-time assignment. By then, our mother had reached the toileting/diaper stage, resulting in zero siblings volunteering for the duty (or doodie?), so I resigned myself to staying home with her. It was the only way I could avoid draining our own family savings and Caitlin's college money. Jinx would have been mortified at either prospect.

My brothers and sister accepted the fact there would be little (if any) money left to split between the four of us at the time of mom's demise. In the end, Jinx *outlived* her savings by one month.

Hands down, being my mother's chief caregiver was the most challenging job of my life, so far, but I cringe whenever somebody refers to me as "a saint" because I know the truth. My seemingly selfless care to her was *not* unconditional. Besides the financial aspect, there were a few other strings attached.

First and foremost, if Jinx had been a danger to my family, she would not have remained with us in our home. A woman in my neighborhood used to relay ongoing horrific tales to me of her demented mother terrorizing her with kitchen knives! What the $%#&!? Lucky for her, she wasn't my mother; I would have shipped her out ANY way I could, including completely surrendering her to the state.

Another condition for care was mom's overall demeanor. If she had been a mean, belligerent, horrible woman, my generosity and compassion would have been short-lived. Ultimately, my family's peace would have taken precedence over my mother's needs, and she would have had to go – especially if she had spewed nasty names or profanity at Caitlin.

Bottom line: If I hadn't *genuinely* loved my mother and felt she had *earned* my care and devotion, I couldn't have done it unbegrudgingly, so I wouldn't have done it at all. It's a *huge* undertaking. From my experience, I believe people who sacrifice everything (mental/physical health and financial stability) in order to care for someone solely out of guilt or obligation are not doing anyone any favors. "Nobody else will take him," and, "I don't like her but she's still my mother," are disastrous reasons for accepting the job. What sick person wants a bitter, resentful nurse?

For all the generous, compassionate souls who find themselves in the all-consuming caregiver role, doing everything you can to remain mentally sharp, physically fit, and fiscally sound will help you stay on top of your game. It's the best way to increase the odds of a more rewarding experience for all concerned. The old adage is true: *Sometimes, the hardest road leads to the most beautiful destination.*

If you're as lucky as I am, you'll discover some unexpected, exquisite benefits on the journey as well. The patience, compassion, and resourcefulness exhibited by my husband and daughter, that I witnessed every single day in their loving care of Jinx, forever changed the way I look at them.

My pride in Caitlin was already quite significant. I don't care how biased it sounds, she's an extraordinary young woman by any measure of the word. But the maturity, and impressive grace-under-pressure she displayed daily, regarding the meticulous care of her grandmother, positively blew me away. She rose to my highest level of awe and respect. Barely out of her teens (and sick, herself), she bravely watched a woman she adored and revered her entire life – someone who had taken care of *her* – gradually transform into a dependent toddler. It was no doubt as unbearable for her as it was me, yet she selflessly kept much of her grief and tears private, so as not to add to my own.

As for Harold, what more can I say about that man's unwavering support and commitment to Jinx (and to me, of course)? Who would've guessed the sight of him kneeling at the feet of an elderly woman, tenderly removing soggy pajama bottoms from her legs, could be one of the sweetest and sexiest sights I've ever seen?

To be sure, my two fellow Musketeers and I were the recipients of gratifying personal growth, in a myriad of ways. We shared a unique, life-affirming experience together; one which enriched us as a family and individually. We were there for *her* and for *each other*. Realizing one's own inner-strength, dedication, tenacity and resiliency builds immense pride and self-confidence, as does rising to the occasion in benevolent servitude to a loved one.

Over the years, since mom's passing, I've been asked many times, "Knowing what you know now – how painfully difficult it is – would you do it again?"

My answer remains resolute, "In a heartbeat."

JINX'S DISNEYLAND BIRTHDAY

What can we do for Mom's 85th birthday?" I pondered almost daily. The milestone occasion, December 4th, was only six weeks away. I wanted to plan something extra-special and super-fun for my mother, while she still had enough cognitive function to enjoy it. It seemed each passing month robbed us of another piece of her. We had no way to estimate when the sand in her mental hourglass would run out, so we needed to seize the day with a memorable (to us, anyway) celebration.

I entertained thoughts of taking mom somewhere, but traveling with her was not an easy task, as I had discovered on our recent summer trip to Colorado. I certainly didn't regret going, but it had left me feeling exhausted, wishing I had had some help. Airports are stressful, confusing places, even *without* having to manage a dementia patient in a wheelchair. Although mom could still walk, the chair was really our only feasible option; her painstakingly, slow shuffle would have been a definite hindrance at *ginormous* Denver International. And don't even get me started on her restroom requirements!

Our Phoenix Sky Harbor Airport security checkpoint experience had to be the most mortifying part of the trip, where to my complete embarrassment, I realized my mother hadn't lost her ingrained, racist suspicion of African Americans. When a black, male TSA agent politely offered to help put her pocketbook on the conveyor belt, she fearfully gripped the bag tightly to her chest with both hands – like a mugging victim

136

– her eyes filling with terror, her head shaking in panic. I lost count of how many times I apologized profusely to the poor man. He seemed unphased, but it still made me cringe. Remembering my struggles at both airports helped me conclude that if I wanted to do a birthday trip with mom, of any kind, I would need to enlist some helpers.

Eventually, the answer came to me when I asked myself, *Where would any kid like to spend their birthday? Disneyland, of course!* Mom hadn't been there since we took her on vacation with us when Caitlin was in kindergarten. I'll never forget how that forever-young, seventy-year-old woman raced around the park, easily keeping pace with her exuberant granddaughter (both having ingested too much sugar!). She had boundless energy, which was extra impressive considering we had spent the previous day traversing SeaWorld from end-to-end!

I knew those days were long gone now, but that didn't deter me. Realistically, this trip would be much different, but I saw no reason it should be any less fun.

Harold, Caitlin, and I decided the long Thanksgiving holiday weekend would work best for our celebratory trip. I also threw the idea out to my siblings, to see if they would be interested in joining us.

I knew Jaime and Billy didn't have the money necessary for the special event, so I made the following offer to them: Mom would fund their complete trips *if* they would act as her escorts. She would ride with *them* for the six-hour drive to and from Arizona and stay with *them* in their hotel room (bedroom for her, pull-out couch for them) all three nights. They would also be the ones *solely* responsible for pushing her wheelchair each day. The guys were immediately on board with my proposal, both chiming in with a resounding, "Hell yeah, we'll go!"

Unfortunately, my sister had her own Disneyland trip planned for the coming weeks, so she declined my invitation. I wish Karen would have postponed hers in favor of ours – it would have been even more fun with her there, since she's the biggest Disney fan in the whole universe (not an exaggeration!).

After making all the arrangements, I suddenly realized I had forgotten to ask the birthday girl how *she* felt about the trip.

"Hey Ma, would you like to go to Disneyland for your birthday? You know, the big park in California where Mickey Mouse lives?"

Without hesitating, mom exclaimed, "Oh boy! You betcha!"

Did she actually know what I was talking about? I don't know. Did she even remember what Disneyland was? Doubtful. But mom definitely knew the famous rodent – from watching Mickey Mouse Clubhouse every morning. Most likely, the excitement in my voice was the primary trigger for her own enthusiastic answer. It didn't matter – the trip was on!

Early Thanksgiving morning, Jaime and Billy arrived at our house to collect mom. They planned to follow behind our car for the trek across the desert to the "Happiest Place on Earth." The drive over to Anaheim, California went smoothly, leaving us with a few hours to kill prior to our dinner reservation at The Rainforest Café. Our hotel was walking distance to the restaurant, located in the Downtown Disneyland District; a lively, outdoor shopping/dining/entertainment complex adjacent to the park which does not require an admission ticket.

Since we all agreed mom definitely needed a special birthday hat, a trip through the Downtown Disney shops topped our agenda. It would also give my brothers a chance to practice wheeling their mother amidst throngs of people – a skill they would absolutely need the following day in the popular park.

Mom wasted no time picking out a hat. Within minutes of entering the first store, her eyes went straight for the bejeweled, neon pink, Minnie

Mouse princess ears, complete with shimmery veil. Well, almost complete – I also had "Jinx" monogrammed on it for her.

Naturally, Princess Jinx became the center of attention at The Rainforest Café, with the waitstaff giving her the royal treatment and fellow diners joining our chorus of "Happy Birthday." It turned out to be the perfect place for our birthday/holiday dinner celebration. The safari-themed restaurant is famous for its life-size, animatronic, jungle animals throughout the dining area. The apes beating on their chests, elephants spraying water, and chimps chattering while we ate made for a wild Thanksgiving gathering, indeed!

The next morning, before heading into Disneyland, we met for a hearty breakfast at a nearby diner. Billy and Jaime got the hilarity rolling with their tales of mom's nighttime escapades. They said she put on a "strip show" by changing into her pajamas with her bedroom window drapes wide-open. When she heard what she'd done, mom laughed so hard she blew orange juice out of her nose, exclaiming "I'm so silly!"

Her sons went on to say how she also wandered out of her room around midnight, not knowing she wasn't at home, looking for the kitchen. Mom cracked up again, "I couldn't find it!" She had always had a wonderful ability to laugh at herself, and it was even more endearing now. I was glad my brothers were getting a chance to experience a taste of our daily life at home with mom – an odd but lovely blend of humor and pathos.

About twenty minutes prior to the gates opening, we eagerly gathered at the main entrance plaza to Disneyland Park. The California sun helped warm us a bit on that brisk, November morning. Excited families clustered around us, bundled in all manner of Disney attire – character sweatshirts, Goofy hats, and Mickey ears – chattering nonstop. As I had expected, the park crowd was still relatively sparse. Black Friday, the mega-shopping day after Thanksgiving, diverts many people to the malls until late afternoon. It was a primary reason of mine for choosing that particular day for our visit.

During our short wait, we decided to plan our "ride strategy." Mom quickly reminded us, "No scary rollercoasters!" We had no intentions of frightening the bejesus out of her, so we promised we wouldn't take her on any. However, the rest of the group unanimously chose park favorite Space Mountain (a rollercoaster in the dark) for our first ride of the day, due to the extremely long lines we'd inevitably encounter later on.

When the Disney "cast members" finally let everybody into the park, the six of us hurried directly to Tomorrowland, the futuristic, space-themed area. Mom's two attendants adeptly maneuvered her wheelchair through already bustling Main Street U.S.A. – her princess veil billowing up behind her in the breeze. Onward to Space Mountain!

Our strategy worked out well: Harold, Caitlin, and I took our turn first, while Billy and Jaime checked out the surrounding space-age sights with mom. Afterwards, the three of us wheeled her around the adjacent giftshop so my brothers could enjoy the raucous rollercoaster. Mom got a kick out of seeing them emerge from the thrill-ride with crazy-looking, wind-blown hair. The Star Tours attraction was right around the corner, so we headed for that, eager for her to join us all on that one.

As we stood in the line for the 3D, flight-simulator ride, I wondered if the realistic journey through the Star Wars galaxy would be too intense and turbulent for mom. Even though the spacecraft doesn't physically leave the "launchpad," the lurching seats jerk you around quite a bit. Images of comets and asteroids barreling toward her could also be quite frightening. It was a crapshoot. Mom said she wanted to go on, but should we have listened to her? Since she no longer possessed enough language to always adequately express her emotions, I had to rely on her face and body language for clues. At that moment, all I had was smiles.

The time had passed for backing out; Caitlin buckled her granny in for her "flight." Mom looked quite calm and cool – seriously rocking her 3-D glasses. I decided to relax and go with it. I was glad I did! I could hear her chuckling throughout the entire ride. She had a blast! When it was over, she was all smiles and said she liked it. Next stop Fantasyland!

As you've probably guessed, our family had an advantage with mom's wheelchair; it significantly reduced our time spent in the otherwise daunting lines, allowing us to get on practically every ride in the park that day. I should clarify by saying people with disabilities don't automatically cut to the front of the line, ahead of everybody else. They must wait their turn in the wheelchair line (which is significantly shorter), where the attendant attempts to equally distribute them amongst the other riders. Mom's chair ensured our wait time, for any ride, never exceeded twenty minutes the entire day!

Some park patrons may feel allowing five, non-disabled people to accompany their relative in the wheelchair line is unfair. Harold definitely felt uncomfortable about it, and I admit we pushed the envelope a bit on its intended purpose. However, our guilt became short-lived once we realized the park was riddled with "wheelchair fakes." They were unashamedly everywhere! We witnessed one old phony, on his motorized, mobility scooter in the disability line for Alice in Wonderland, striding up a hilly area a short time later, on two perfectly strong legs – carrying a tray laden with food and drinks!

Our family wasn't trying to cash-in on mom's disability, we merely shared one common goal: We all sincerely wanted to enjoy each attraction beside the birthday girl, so we could experience the wonder through *her* eyes. After all, that was the purpose of the trip.

Everywhere we went, birthday wishes, and congratulations followed, as people learned of Jinx's impending 85th. I think our mother actually started to believe she was a true princess, especially with her two doting "coachmen" pushing her "imperial carriage" and catering to her every wish. Mom was having a real, royal ball!

During our trip through Fantasyland, mom munched on churros and sipped lemonade. She soared on Dumbo (the flying elephant ride), rode King Arthur's Carousel, and delighted in Peter Pan's Flight. Sailing high over London to Neverland in a pirate galleon, mom joyously proclaimed, "Hey, I can fly!" and "I see an alligator down there!"

Gauging mom's level of enjoyment on a ride wasn't always an easy call for me. Her owl-eyed look of wonder and her owl-eyed look of fright were pretty much the same. While on It's a Small World, we found it very hard to discern the difference. Sometimes, during the slow-moving boat ride, she appeared downright disturbed by the international, singing dolls and animals (lip-syncing llamas can be creepy!), and other times she merrily sang along with the repetitive, catchy tune – "…it's a small world after all."

In Adventureland, mom seemed to enjoy the Jungle Cruise riverboat ride, for the most part. She laughed and pointed at the frolicking elephants and hippos rising out of the water but shuddered at the sight of the king cobras and hyenas. I wish we could have also taken her into Tarzan's Treehouse, the attraction next door, but it can only be reached by those able to climb continuous, winding stairs up an 80-foot-tall tree. Pass on that one! Instead, we headed straight to Indiana Jones Adventure.

By far, the decision to allow mom on that ride proved to be my most egregious faux pas of the day. My poor mother must have been terrified out of her mind. As soon as the ride started, I knew I had had a serious lapse in judgment. Perhaps mom's enjoyment of Star Tours lulled me into a false sense of confidence.

It may not be a "scary rollercoaster," but it *is* a fast-paced thrill ride; one which simulates a jeep driving over rough terrain, collapsing bridges, and molten lava! The perilous expedition takes place inside a cursed, crumbling temple and includes encounters with slithering snakes, swarms of giant bugs, and screaming mummies. Riders also hear and feel the breeze of poison blow darts and spears whizzing past their heads. Lastly, an oncoming massive boulder rolls directly into the jeep's path. What in the world was I thinking?!

Throughout the ride, I watched mom's face contort with fright. Clearly horrified, she tightly hung onto the bar in front of her with both hands and stiffened arms. She never made a single sound and didn't become distraught or hysterical, but she was obviously very scared. I couldn't believe I had subjected my mother to snakes and bugs – the two things she feared most on earth (with the possible exception of black TSA agents). After we got off, I tried to lighten the mood by jokingly asking if she'd like to go on that ride again, to which she vigorously shook her head and replied, "I don't think so!"

As not only her daughter, but primary caregiver, the blame was mine alone to bear. The upsetting experience could have turned out much worse and made me suddenly realize I had not given enough *serious* consideration to mom's overall ability to distinguish fantasy from reality. I knew her better than anybody, and I had failed to properly consider her possible anxiety level. Disneyland is an incredible world of make-believe with much more than wand-waving fairy godmothers, beautiful princesses, and talking animals. The place is loaded with scary imagery; ghosts, pirates, wicked queens, dragons, witches, and even an abominable snow monster lurking in the Matterhorn (no, Jinx did not ride that one!). I wondered exactly how mom's brain processed such otherworldly sights. People with Alzheimer's live in the present moment and take things quite literally. Thankfully, mom would have no memory of her awful "adventure."

We all decided a long, leisurely break was in order. Throughout the day, we had made plenty of restroom pit stops and taken short breathers, mostly for mom's sake, but now the situation called for a major rest. Everyone agreed Frontierland's Golden Horseshoe Saloon would be the perfect place to reenergize; we could eat ice cream sundaes and watch the musical, holiday stage show starring "Billy Hill and the Hillbillies." The talented bunch of comedic fiddlers had us all knee-slapping and toe-tapping for an hour. After the western show ended, we were lucky enough to happen upon a lively, musical performance in New Orleans Square, where a swinging jazz band had the crowd boogieing to "Sweet Georgia Brown."

Hands down, mom's favorite attraction in the whole park was the Enchanted Tiki Room. The tiny Polynesian "theater in the round" showcases over 200 choreographed, animatronic, tropical birds, wooden tiki gods, and colorful flowers performing songs and comedy. A quartet of internationally diverse macaws – José, Michael, Pierre, and Fritz – lead the show. Their bright feathers match the colors of their home flags, Mexico, Ireland, France, and Germany, respectively. For added hilarity, each one has an exaggerated foreign accent. Their silly bird banter was quite a hoot (bad pun intended):

José: "My siestas are getting 'chorter and 'chorter."

Fritz: "Ach du liebe! I almost fell off my perch!"

The crazy parrots tickled mom to no end. I'd say the Tiki Room definitely enchanted her! She even sang along to one of the show's songs, amazingly remembering it from her own childhood.

"Let's all sing like the birdies sing...tweet, tweet-tweet, tweet-tweet!"

Previously unbeknownst to me, the Enchanted Tiki Room has a self-service, wheelchair lift for access. I hadn't realized it until Jaime and Billy suddenly popped into the theater from a different entrance. The reason I hadn't noticed the mini-elevator for mom was because *I didn't need to*. My sweet brothers took care of everything! I have to say, inviting those two guys on the trip was a stroke of brilliance on my part. They made the entire trip WAY more fun and enabled Harold, Caitlin, and I to take a much-needed break from our regular duties. They floored me with their tireless devotion to our mother. I couldn't have asked for more diligent, joyous, tender-loving attendants.

As dusk settled over Disneyland, hundreds of thousands of holiday lights began to pop on all over the park – transforming it into a dazzling wonderland of festive color. According to mom, it looked like "a sparkly, sugar cookie." Her face glowed in the illumination, as we eagerly awaited the Christmas Fantasy Parade. Again, mom's wheelchair worked to our benefit – allowing us special access to a prime viewing spot along the Main Street parade route.

We could hear the jubilant music of the parade before we could see it, but soon the procession of two-story-high, whimsical floats lumbered into view, flanked by giant toy soldiers, and whirling Disney princesses. Utterly captivated, mom excitedly (and accurately) yelled out the names and actions of familiar Disney characters as they went by.

"Winnie the Pooh sleigh-riding!"

"Goofy making gingerbread!"

"Beauty and the Beast dancing!"

And last but never least, "There's Santa Claus!"

I blinked away tears, remembering our toddler Caitlin — at the parade two decades earlier — sounding quite similar, perched high atop her papa's shoulders. Where had the time gone?

The magnificent parade would have been a wonderful way to end our glorious Disney day, but incredibly, there was still more in store for our senses: A spectacular fireworks display, which included a dramatic musical light show projected onto Sleeping Beauty's Castle and the Main Street storefronts. Mom audibly gasped with delight each time the castle changed a different color in sync to orchestral music. A dazzling flight by Tinker Bell (Peter Pan's sassy fairy friend), from the peak of the Matterhorn, over to the highest turret of the castle, capped off the extravaganza and signaled the finale — a lovely holiday snowfall.

Standing in the middle of Main Street, U.S.A., I looked over at the elated faces of my two brothers, my husband, daughter, and mother — all of them gazing up into the moonlit sky at the soft snowflakes drifting down onto their heads. We were all entranced in that moment together, under the spell of Disney magic. I gave my mother's mittened hand a tender squeeze and tried to commit the beauty of her joyous face to memory; the wondrous expression of a child on Christmas morning. I was desperate to absorb every tiny detail and nuance of her face, in the hope of forever capturing the sublime image and moment in time — a moment which my aching heart knew would never come again.

As the show came to an end, the mesmerized crowd dispersed, slowly in all directions. Although the park wouldn't be closing for another hour or two, our exhausted little group ambled down the middle of Main Street toward the exit turnstiles; ten o'clock was plenty late enough for everyone. Plus, nothing could top the mind-blowing pyrotechnics and pageantry we had just witnessed — truly a magical ending to a magical day.

"You ready to go, birthday girl?" I asked mom, while tucking her wool scarf into her coat and her blanket tighter around her legs. The autumn night had gotten quite chilly.

She nodded and yawned, "Yeah, I'm tired."

It was past bedtime now, for everybody's favorite princess.

Mom's shimmery, silver veil fluttered behind her in the night breeze as Jaime and Billy wheeled her past the illuminated giftshop windows. At the Town Square, we stopped and turned, for one last look – a final mental snapshot – at the iconic blue and pink castle glittering at the opposite end of the park.

The walk back to our nearby hotel seemed way longer than its actual time of twenty-minutes. Besides our leg-muscle fatigue, heavy emotions hovered over our family in the brisk evening air, an extraordinary mix of both melancholy and gratification. None of us had held any false illusions; we knew we could never give mom an *unforgettable* experience, or a trip she'd *always remember*. But mom's birthday celebration was a triumph, nevertheless, deserving of our sense of achievement and self-satisfaction. Our family had fully succeeded in giving her an amazing time *while* it was happening; a time none of us would *ever* forget.

We also knew that perfect part of the trip was over, and the six of us would be parting ways the following morning: Harold, Caitlin, and I would be heading 100 miles south to San Diego for some sailing, so Billy and Jaime could enjoy extra time alone with their beloved mother, for what would ultimately be her final stroll along the ocean in Newport Beach, arm-in-arm with her two boys.

At the hotel lobby, we said our goodnights and agreed upon a later hour to meet for breakfast; there would be no early-risers tomorrow morning. We were all beat. I gave mom a long hug and a loud smooch before Caitlin cut in for a hug of her own.

"Was that the BEST birthday you ever had, Grandma?"

Through her sleepy smile, mom managed a faint but heartfelt, "You betcha!"

…and that was good enough for us.

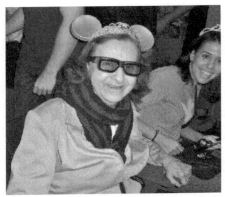

Mom & Caitlin on Star Tours ride at Disneyland

THE QUEEN'S SPEECH

Despite the entire Scribner clan hailing from New Jersey, none of us acquired the Joe Pesci, *My Cousin Vinnie* accent except for Jinx. Decades before her language dissipated due to Alzheimer's, mom's way of speaking was not always easily understood – even by her own family members.

One of the most mysterious terms I recall my mother using, during my childhood, was "toe pat." Whenever I asked her what a "toe pat" was, she'd only say it was where she took walks by the canal when she was a kid, with no further explanation. Naturally, I would try to picture in my mind what a "toe pat" might be, but all I could come up with was an image of barefoot kids tiptoeing around some water.

Believe it or not, I was left in the dark on this matter well into my thirty's. One day, out of the blue, I realized that despite living in Arizona for twenty years, mom still maintained one aspect of her New Jersey accent. She omitted the "h" in many of her words, thus her vernacular included the following pronunciations: "toot'brush," "birt'day," "sout'west," and just like *Cousin Vinny* – "yout's."

It was during this mental inventory of my mother's vocabulary that the meaning of "toe pat" finally dawned on me. "Toe pat" was *towpath*; a path beside an inland waterway used for towing boats. Mystery finally solved! Mom had taken walks along the *towpaths* of the Jersey canals when she was a kid! It's hard to believe something so obvious had perplexed me for so long.

My sudden realization about mom's speech pattern didn't automatically put an end to the ongoing miscommunication between the two of us. I remember another bit of bafflement I had on a trip to K-Mart when my mother said to me, "Remind me to take a look at some 'clawt' while we're in here."

"You want to look at some *clawt*?" I had no idea what she was talking about.

"Yeah, you know…CLAWT!" She figured saying it louder would help clarify.

Only when she put the word into context, did I finally understand what she meant.

"I need some *clawt* to make a dress for Caitlin."

"Oh, cloth! You want to buy fabric!"

Evidently, I was a slow learner when it came to mastering "Jersey-speak," but I wasn't the only one. Poor Caitlin is also still embarrassed about her own ignorance. She was 10-years-old before she realized "the forcha-jul-eye" her grandmother spoke of was actually a date on the calendar – the *fourth* of July – Independence Day. Every year, she and I still wish each other "Happy Forcha-jul-eye!"

Through a lovely stroke of serendipity, during my mother's cognitive decline, I happened to be working on a speech-language pathology degree. The subject matter of how we acquire language skills had always been of special interest to me, but I had no idea when I began my studies how much it would help me in my role as mom's caregiver, especially once her ability to communicate started to disintegrate.

A year or so after resigning from my full-time teaching position, I enrolled in an online speech-therapy degree program. Submerging myself in a new field of study provided a mental distraction from my mother's illness.

Additionally, as mom's care required me to be home with her more, the online classes became a lifeline to the outside, professional world without having to physically leave the house.

From the onset of Jinx's dementia, I knew she would eventually lose her ability to speak, but I hadn't really envisioned *exactly* how that would manifest itself. There were so many other seemingly more critical issues when it came to my mother's care, her language skills became a low-priority problem; one for the back burner. I guess I imagined she would just abruptly stop talking one day, but it turned out to be far more complicated and became one of my biggest challenges.

Jinx was losing her ability to *process language*, which meant her entire communication system was breaking down; both the comprehension of words spoken to her and the verbal expression of her own thoughts. Initially, before I began my related studies, her language *appeared* to be deteriorating in an unpredictable manner, leaving us bewildered about the best way to communicate with her. The following is a perfect example:

One day, in the early stages of mom's illness, I realized she wasn't changing her underwear anymore; her bras and panties were AWOL from the laundry basket. When I brought this to her attention, she shrugged it off with her usual self-deprecating humor, "I guess I'm losing my marbles again!" Then she'd promptly correct the behavior for a few days before eventually returning to it again. The purchase of an inexpensive hook rack seemed to solve the problem. I attached it to her bedroom door, labeled the hooks Sunday-Saturday, and hung clean undergarments from each one. *There, that should take care of it!*

The system worked very well for a month or two before my mother began wearing the same underwear again every day. Verbal reminders became useless. As did the large whiteboard I had fastened to her bedroom

151

closet which read, "DON'T FORGET TO PUT ON CLEAN UNDERPANTS!" in giant red letters.

I tore down the sign and the hooks in frustration, as I did later on with my "Flush Your Toilet Paper!" poster when it had failed to change mom's behavior. Expending so much mental energy on a problem, with no real permanent solution, was exhausting. I resigned myself to physically supervising my mother – like a prison guard – to ensure she put on clean clothes every day.

If only I would have been armed with my speech knowledge earlier in the game, it would have saved me a whole lot of grief. The memory reminders I used on mom were all viable ideas, but they would have been far more effective had they been implemented in accordance with mom's *receptive language* ability. Before I learned how to better identify what her ability actually was, my own communication efforts often failed, out of ignorance.

Allow me to share a bit of speech-language background I gleaned from my classes. Throughout this chapter and the one that follows, I will refer to information from the American Speech-Language-Hearing Association (ASHA) website, as well as a textbook from one of my courses: Born to Talk an Introduction to Speech and Language Development, by Merle R. Howard and Lloyd M. Hulit. My instructor's lessons (also one of my sources) were derived from the same text.

The following two concepts and definitions are essential in understanding my mother's deteriorating communication.

> **Receptive Language** is the understanding of language "input;" of information received, which includes the words (written or spoken) and gestures of others. It also involves the ability to interpret a question as a question.
>
> **Expressive Language** is the "output" of language; being able to put our thoughts and needs into words that make sense and are grammatically correct. It should not be confused with the mechanics of speech production – which is how we make sounds using our lips, tongue, teeth, and other parts of the mouth.

I wasted a lot of time and energy on signage my mother couldn't understand. Mom's ability to read (receptive language) the words on a sign didn't equal comprehension. I should have remembered that from all of the Structured English Immersion students I taught over the years. Many of them could read a passage from a science textbook aloud to me perfectly, but they had no idea what the words meant. Perhaps, the words "clean underpants" no longer had any meaning at all to mom, which would explain why the matter didn't seem to concern her.

Once I realized mom could not properly process language anymore, I stopped spinning my wheels in futility. Still, I wondered if there was a way to second-guess or anticipate her communication ability, so I could adjust my expectations accordingly. There didn't seem to be any predictability to her language decline. And then it dawned on me – there was an obvious and profound pattern.

From birth through childhood we acquire language in stages; in a specific *sequential, predictable* order. For example: A typical two-year-old has a vocabulary of 200-300 words and uses 3-4 word sentences. However, if a middle schooler possessed such limited language skills, there would most likely be something developmentally wrong.

Since the onset of her dementia, I had been witnessing my mother literally aging backward. It suddenly occurred to me she was losing her ability to communicate in the *reverse sequential order* by which she acquired it — an order which would also have to be predictable.

What an eye-opener! Once I recognized what was happening to mom, I could easily refer to the stages of language development in children and follow them backward. Eliminating the unpredictability consequently reduced much of my frustration in communicating with her. It also provided me with another immensely helpful benefit; it enabled me to easily estimate Jinx's approximate mental age. For example, the fact mom could no longer understand non-literal language, such as sarcasm, irony, hyperbole, or rhetorical questions, was a sure sign she had fallen below the cognitive age of ten, since that's when we typically acquire that language skill.

If only I could have gotten my husband to take my newfound knowledge seriously. Despite many attempts to enlighten Harold on the subject of mom's loss of language processing, he continued to kid and tease his demented mother-in-law in the good-natured way he had done throughout most of our marriage. We'd no sooner sit down to dinner, when he'd make some goofy remark like, "What's the matter Jinx? Are you getting too lazy to cook us dinner in your old age?" prompting her to stop and glare at him for a few seconds, while she pondered a verbal response. With few words at her disposal, she'd stick out her tongue, and give him "the old Bronx cheer," otherwise known as blowing a raspberry.

To which I would always add, "I agree with you, Ma!"

The first time I heard my mother use *immediate echolalia,* a form of parroting used by young children, I was quite taken aback, having recognized it as a speech pattern little kids typically outgrow before they are three-years-old. Our conversation sounded something like this:

Me: "Ma, are you hungry?"

Mom: "Hungry."

Me: "Do you want some lunch?"

Mom: "Lunch."

Me: "Do you want a sandwich?"

Mom: "Sandwich."

Me: "How about pizza?"

Mom: "Pizza."

Sadly, for mom, it meant another step backward on the development chart. Her ability to verbally express her own needs and wants was dwindling. Identifying her approximate age and language problem didn't automatically make me a mind-reader. How was I supposed to know what she wanted to eat, or if she was actually hungry? I figured I'd try *showing* her what food was available and letting her choose.

During mealtimes, I started taking my mother on mini tours of our kitchen – from cupboard to refrigerator, over to the pantry, and back to the refrigerator. She seemed to think it was a game and usually selected nothing. My plan didn't work because it didn't stop the parroting.

Me: "We have tomato soup and noodle soup..."

Mom: "Soup."

Me: "We have leftover chicken..."

Mom: "Chicken."

I soon gave up on offering her options and decided to make life simpler for myself – I made whatever I thought she'd enjoy and served it to her.

During this time period (about five years into her dementia), I remember contemplating, "Has my mother's language really been reduced to less than a three-year-old's?" It was so difficult for me to fathom my mother as a preschooler. I needed to test my theory.

My speech-therapy teacher granted me permission to use Jinx (rather than a child) as my case study for a few class assignments. The first one required me to design an expressive language lesson geared for kindergarten to second grade. I couldn't wait to try the activity I created with my mother.

The lesson involved grouping twenty, small, plastic, animals by their commonalities and differences, such as where they live (zoo, farm, ocean), or their number of legs. I chose very basic animals for the lesson, such as a horse, fish, lion, and monkey.

First, I told mom to name as many of the animals as she could. She identified only three out of the twenty – the pig, horse and cow. Then I had her name any other types of animals she could think of and she said, "Cat and dog." When I asked her where the animals live, she replied, "In a house." None of the plastic animals were house animals but, of course, a cat and a dog both are, so that response didn't seem too off-base to me. Mom's answer to my next question, "What kind of animal would make a good house pet?" was a different story...

She responded with, "A whale."

So much for kindergarten! Even a 5-year-old knows a whale doesn't live in a house. The activity left me completely stunned. Despite my mother talking to us every day, I really had no idea she couldn't name ten animals. As the lesson continued, mom didn't even know what an ocean, farm, or a zoo was, despite me pointing to photos of them. Finally, when I tried to get her to group the animals by their number of legs (2, 4, or 0), she couldn't. I pondered the gravity of that. There was nothing abstract about how many legs an animal had, since mom could physically see them on each toy. She could see their legs, but she couldn't count them or even recognize the fish had *no* legs. *Holy cow! What does this mean? Was her mental age less than three?*

CALCULATING MOM'S MENTAL AGE

I didn't have to wonder for very long. Coincidentally, the following week's speech lesson had the precise information I was looking for. Specifically, it was about how to calculate the *mean length of utterance* (MLU) from a language sample.

An Utterance is an uninterrupted chain of language.

Mean Length of Utterance (MLU) refers to the average length of each phrase a person uses.

Calculating a child's MLU is a method speech therapists use to determine if their language is within the developmental expectations for their age. With mom as my case study again, I'd be able to match her MLU to a developmental stage and a corresponding age.

The lesson's assignment required a video of mom's language sample (her utterances), which I made via my laptop. Before we began, I asked my mother if she would please help me with my homework assignment, to which she readily agreed, "Yeah, sure!"

For the video session, mom and I sat side-by-side on the couch with one of Caitlin's over-size storybooks propped open between our laps – one containing whimsical illustrations and classic tales such as *The Gingerbread Man* and *The Little Red Hen*. With each turn of the page, I posed a question to my mother about a specific picture such as, "What is this lady making?"; "Where is this girl?"; "Why is this man sad?"

Mom responded with mostly correct answers (aka utterances) such as, "curtains," "kitchen," and "crying," respectively. In all, I asked her twenty-eight questions about the pictures, and she provided twenty-eight answers (utterances).

The correctness of her answer had no bearing on her score. Mom's limited vocabulary was also not the main issue: She identified a fox as a "dog," porridge as "soup," and the measles as "polka dots." The *length* of each phrase or sentence was all that counted. But I couldn't merely count the number of words she spoke; estimating mom's mental age involved counting the number of *morphemes* she used, which is a little trickier. Again, I'll refer to Born to Talk.

What is a Morpheme?

A Morpheme is the smallest unit of language to have meaning, which cannot be further divided.

Example1: The word "pickle" consists of one morpheme; it cannot be divided further. The word "pickles" consists of two morphemes – "pickle" plus the suffix "s" – which changes the meaning of the word by making it plural.

Example2: The word "talk" consists of one morpheme; it cannot be divided further. The word "talked" consists of two morphemes – "talk" plus the suffix "ed" – which changes the meaning of the word by making it past tense.

My mother's longest answer was "Trying to put on a pair of socks." The sentence has 8 words but 10 *morphemes*. The suffix "ing" added to "try" expands the meaning of the word, as does the "s" on the end of "socks." Thus, the more morphemes an utterance has, the more meaning it has, resulting in a higher score.

After recording our video session, it was time to calculate Jinx's *Mean Length of Utterance* (MLU), the score that would determine mom's approximate mental age:

How to Calculate MLU

1. I transcribed each of mom's 28 utterances from the video, and listed them on the Language Sample Form

2. I counted the morphemes in each utterance and entered the data in the form accordingly

3. I divided the total number of morphemes (68) by the total of utterances (28)

4. $68/28 = 2.4$

5. An MLU score of 2.4 meant the average length of mom's utterances was 2.4 morphemes.

6. I plugged the MLU score of 2.4 into the "Stages of Development" chart.

7. 2.4 falls within Stage II on the chart, for an approximate age range of 2-2½ years

---

The Stage Two Language Characteristics fit her perfectly (see guide). It definitely explained why she was parroting me so much – my mother possessed the expressive language of a two-and-a-half-year-old child.

I sat solemnly at the kitchen table, studying mom's data spread out before me, and tried wrapping my brain around it. I clicked on the six-minute-long video of the two of us with the storybook and watched it again; this time through the emotional eyes of a daughter, rather than a speech-therapy student. It was incredibly touching, and I immediately treasured it.

I moved to the family room and snuggled next to my mother on the couch, giving her a tight, lingering hug.

"Thanks for helping me with my homework, Ma. I got an 'A' on it!" (of course, I hadn't even submitted it to the instructor yet)

Mom smiled proudly at me and replied, "Oh good.................What homework?"

The video I made that day turned out to be invaluable to our family. It's the last recording of Jinx speaking.

As I reflected on my mother's language score, I knew it made perfect sense; mom rarely expressed more than two words at a time. It was no real surprise it matched the age of a toddler; everything else about her did too. I certainly felt like the mother of a two-year-old: I bathed her, dressed her, toileted her, and played with her. Our days were filled with coloring pictures, blowing bubbles on the porch swing, putting preschool jigsaw puzzles together, and watching cartoons on TV. I refused to allow myself to dwell on the obvious heartbreaking difference: A toddler's future is normally a bright one, filled with promise and hope.

I had to admit, I ached to hear mom's Jersey-speak once again, but her humorous *My Cousin Vinnie* lingo was long gone. I knew the total loss of her language loomed right around the corner.

Calculating Mean Length of Utterance Table

	Jinx's Utterances	Morphemes
1.	Apron	1
2.	Gingerbread	2
3.	Running	2
4.	A Cow	2
5.	Baking	2
6.	Kitchen	1
7.	I Don't Know	4
8.	Dog	1
9.	Horse	1
10.	Gray	1
11.	Thinking of Jumping in the Water	8
12.	Troll	1
13.	Trying to Put on a Pair of Socks	10
14.	Pig	1
15.	Old Man	2
16.	Crying	2
17.	No	1
18.	I Don't Know	4
19.	Sewing	2
20.	Curtains	2
21.	Pig	1
22.	I Don't Know	4
23.	Sick	1
23.	Polka Dots	3
25.	Big Mess	2
26.	Candy	1
27.	She Don't Like It	5
28	Soup	1
	Total Morphemes:	68
	68 Morphemes ÷ 28 Utterances = MLU	2.4

Language Characteristics Guide
STAGE 2

- 27-30 months of age
- MLU score 2.0-2.5
- "ed" an "ing" suffixes
- Plurals
- Overgeneralization of verb and plural endings
- Pronouns – him/her, hims/hers
- Questions by intonation and WH (what, where, who, why, when/how) questions

- 400-word vocabulary
- Politeness markers – please and thank you
- Emotional understanding

TIME FOR A NURSING HOME?
(Applying for State Assistance)

How do we know when it's time to move mom to a skilled nursing home?

It was one of the toughest questions I had to maintain on the backburner of my brain during all the years as Jinx's caregiver. I had given it a lot of serious consideration and knew I needed to take action *before* a crisis arose. Alzheimer's symptoms and complications rarely give notice; they have a lousy way of suddenly appearing out of leftfield.

The proverbial "line in the sand" had been drawn in my mind for quite some time. When mom's medical needs surpassed my family's scope of knowledge and abilities, it would no longer be in her best interest to live at home anymore. We couldn't allow her health and safety to be compromised by our ignorance. Mom's needs were well-past that of an assisted-living or memory care facility, so she would need a skilled nursing home.

I had hoped by the time that day arrived, Jinx would have lost the ability to recognize us as her immediate family, and our house as her home, would already be gone. I still feared the heartbreaking scenario if that were not the case: My mother – aka my little girl – crying her eyes out, pleading for us to let her stay. She wouldn't have the mental capacity to understand what she could only perceive as an extreme punishment.

In the spring of 2013 (about a year before my mother's passing), I accurately predicted a nursing home would become necessary within the next six months. The criteria had been met, so it was definitely on the horizon. Mom's recently diagnosed congestive heart failure symptoms were already beyond my comfort zone.

Jinx's high blood pressure required daily monitoring and medication. The ineffective pumping of her heart caused her ankles and feet to swell, which required a diuretic to relieve the fluid retention. Consequently, the diuretic resulted in hourly diaper changes. Soggy diapers led to urinary tract infections, which required more doctor visits and antibiotic prescriptions. My mother's never-ending cycle of complications, coupled with her ever-worsening dementia, turned out to be the final straw.

I'm in over my head now. I'm not a goddamn nurse!

If all that wasn't overwhelming enough, my mother's shuffling gait was causing her to trip and stumble with greater frequency. The entire downstairs level of our house – mom's living area – has flagstone flooring. Its uneven surface presented a hazard for her slippered feet. A tragic fall seemed inevitable.

Although Jinx had a cane, she no longer understood how to use it for balance – she hung it off her forearm, so it didn't even touch the ground. Mom looked cute as could be carrying the cane on her elbow, like a pocketbook, but it had to be just a matter of time before she took a nose-dive into the stone floor. I had a dreaded suspicion my mother probably only had about six more months of being able to walk *at all*.

How would I care for her then? How would I lift her when nobody else was home?

It was time to begin the process of arranging for alternative nursing care. I already knew my mother's Medicare wasn't going to pay for anyone to come to the house and help me. My online research uncovered only one promising option for mom: State financial assistance. Jinx's paltry income of $1,200 per month, lack of assets, and need for ongoing care, stood to qualify her for subsidized nursing care via Arizona's Medicaid program,

164

Arizona Long Term Care System (ALTCS). Every state has some version of this. The website stated the application process took approximately 90 days, so I knew I needed to get the ball rolling promptly. It also listed the following criteria for qualification of state aid:

1. Two Major Components to the Application Process
   a. Financial Assessment
   b. Functional/Medical Assessment
2. Monthly Income Limit is $2,100
3. Countable Resources (Bank Accounts, Insurance Policies) Limit is $2,000

I figured mom would easily ace the functional/medical assessment. The mandatory in-home visit would irrefutably prove my mother's obvious need for full-time care. I also wasn't worried about her monthly income, which fell well below the ALTCS limit. The only possible fly in the ointment was the money I had moved from mom's CD account into the "holding account," from which I drew my caregiver salary. It was no longer a sizable sum, but it was still significantly more than the state's allowable amount for countable resources. Plus, it was easily trackable, so I worried about it possibly disqualifying mom.

What do I do if I can't get financial assistance for her? Nursing homes cost upwards of $3,000 a month. Mom can't afford that, and neither can we!

I had a foreboding sense the bureaucratic process for obtaining state assistance was going to be an arduous uphill battle. It was certain to be extremely time-consuming – gathering years' worth of financial documentation as evidence. No doubt they'd make me jump through many pointless hoops for the money. Regardless, I had to bite the bullet and do it. I was at their mercy. I psychologically braced myself for an aggravating experience.

Ultimately, I have to say, I was never happier and more relieved to be proven wrong. Despite my lack of religious beliefs, the two amazing women assigned to my mother's ALTCS case suddenly had me believing in the existence of angels!

The first heaven-sent individual was Carol, the medical assessor who came out to interview my mother and verify her inability to care for herself. I took an instant liking to Carol's plucky personality. We exchanged pleasantries as I led her downstairs to the family room to meet mom, who was sitting silently on the couch, staring straight ahead at a *blank* television screen.

"Are you watching that same show again, Ma?" I laughed. "Aren't you tired of that one yet? Want me to put on Shirley Temple for you?"

"No," she mumbled, too transfixed by her own reflection to notice the stranger in the room.

"There's someone here to meet you, Mom. Carol, this is my mother Josephine Scribner, but everyone calls her Jinx. Ma, this is my friend, Carol."

Carol smiled warmly as she leaned in to shake mom's hand.

"Hi Jinx, it's very nice to meet you. How are you doing today?"

My mother remained seated on the couch but turned briefly to smile at Carol. Clenched horizontally in her mouth, like a dog bone, was her plastic hair comb.

"Okay," she muttered through her teeth. Then she returned her attention back to her "TV program," the comb still secured between her lips.

What happened next caught me totally off-guard: Carol slipped her notebook back into her satchel and placed a consoling hand on my shoulder – as if to prepare me for solemn news.

"And that concludes the interview," she laughed.

I was completely stunned. Mom's entire evaluation was finished in a span of two minutes – no hoops, no red tape, no bullshit. Just one wise, compassionate soul. *Thank you, dear Carol.*

The second angel arrived in the form of Joyce, the financial assessor, who, with the exception of one face-to-face meeting, I dealt with exclusively by phone. Her professionalism and intellect afforded me a much-unexpected peace of mind. But what struck me most about Joyce was her deep, genuine sense of empathy. To my relief, I wasn't dealing with an unfeeling, robotic state worker in a cubicle. She seemed to sincerely care about helping my mother and me. Joyce eventually revealed she'd been in my shoes, as a caregiver herself, to a parent with dementia.

During our initial conversation, I provided an honest and detailed accounting of Jinx's money, including the transfer of her savings to pay myself. I explained I had several years' worth of invoices documenting the amounts. Joyce's first instruction to me was to mail a copy of my mother's estate-planning trust and living will to her, along with mom's most recent bank statement, and my caregiver salary invoices. Easy enough!

About two weeks later, Joyce called back with some disappointing news: The invoices I sent her were useless. The caregiver salary I paid myself could not be counted as a legal expense for mom unless I had a signed, written agreement with her. I informed Joyce that although I had financial and medical power of attorney, I had nothing in writing giving me permission for payment of services.

Joyce was undeterred by my admission. She assured me my mother would qualify for assistance anyway. "Your mother has a meager income of $1,200 a month. She obviously cannot afford a nursing home on that. What I need from you this time is a copy of Josephine's next checking account statement with receipts matching her expenses for food, prescriptions, and anything medical. But instead of documentation for caregiving, I want invoices showing she paid rent and utilities."

"You only need one months' worth of accounting for evidence?" I found it hard to believe.

"Yes," she reassured me once again. "Your mother's application will be approved. I don't want you to worry about it."

Again I was skeptical. "What about the money I transferred from her savings? Don't I still have to account for that?"

"No, and the details will not be investigated," she patiently explained. "Your mother's trust lists no *specific dollar amount* nor banking accounts. In fact, no actual assets are mentioned at all in her legal documents. It clearly stipulates that all moneys and personal items are to be evenly split between her four children. Jinx's savings paid for her care. That's between you and your family."

"And now you, Joyce..."

"What I know is this Mrs. Jaxon: Your mother put *you* in charge of her estate because she knew you would do everything in her best interest, which you obviously have. You saved the state of Arizona untold dollars by caring for your mom all these years. You'll be hearing from me the first week of September, at which time I will formally approve your mother's application for state aid."

I tearfully and profusely thanked Joyce, probably to the point of embarrassment for both of us.

I'll never know what I did to deserve the exceptional kindness extended to me by those two gems – Carol and Joyce. Whether or not either one broke agency protocol to help me, I have no idea, since I'm unable to compare my experience with that of anybody else's. All I know for sure is the stress involved in the daunting first step of moving my mother to a nursing home was considerably lessened by the benevolence and compassionate sensibility of those two extraordinary, unforgettable women. Words alone can't convey the respect and gratitude I will *forever* hold in my heart for them. They are rare souls indeed.

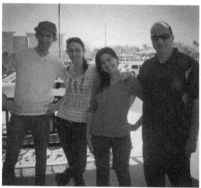

Four of Jinx's grandkids – Michael, Stacy, Caitlin, & Shawn

UNEXPECTED HOSPICE HELP

The next three months were bound to go by slowly, awaiting final approval of mom's state aid. My concern was not over whether she qualified; Joyce had assured me she would. I worried about the prospect of my mother needing full-time nursing care before then. What would I do if she did? I couldn't ignore that very real, unnerving possibility, and I had no game plan other than keeping my fingers crossed.

The summer was already off to a rough start, with mom's congestive heart failure symptoms adding complicated medical duties to my plate. Did I mention I wasn't a nurse? The overwhelming situation left me with a deep sense of despair and weariness. I held no expectation or hope of taking a sailing retreat before September.

Out of the blue, my brother Jaime changed EVERYTHING with one tiny, but impactful, suggestion.

Despite his physically demanding job, my gracious brother faithfully took time at the end of each workday to communicate with me, offering a compassionate nonjudgmental lifeline. The value of having a person to rant to (even if it's electronically) should not be underestimated. Normally, I tried to be more upbeat and sensitive to him, after all, he was losing his mother too. And even though he didn't have to witness her day-to-day decline, he also didn't have the privilege of sharing in her daily joy the way I did.

My email must have sounded *really* bleak to him because it prompted his immediate phone call.

"Marlene, mom's health problems are way more complex now. I think they're severe enough that hospice might come in and help you."

"Doesn't the person have to be on the verge of dying?" I asked.

"Not necessarily. They took care of my friend's grandmother for quite a few months before she passed away. You should call them. It can't hurt to ask."

Holy cow! I wondered if it was indeed true. The next day, I called my daughter's friend Fran, a seasoned nurse (practicing almost 50 years), who confirmed my brother was correct.

"Yes, call them, honey! Hospice will help you."

Before hanging up, Fran gave me a brutally honest piece of advice I deeply appreciated and never forgot:

"Honey, listen to me carefully now…I'm gonna tell you something very important: If your mother starts to fall at any time while you're helping her – in the tub or whatever – JUST LET HER GO! Please do not try to catch her. You're not trained to do so, like I am. Her dead weight will cause you a permanent injury. I know your natural reflex will be to try to catch her, but please don't do it."

Her warning seemed a bit unorthodox to me – maybe even unethical – coming from a healthcare professional. I had to admit it made sense. My automatic reaction would be to try to catch my mother – but self-preservation also came naturally to me – so I promised myself I'd jump out of the way if necessary.

As soon as I hung up from Fran, I called Hospice of the Valley (the leading provider of hospice care in Arizona) to schedule an appointment. A couple of days later, a hospice coordinator named Gail, came to our house to meet with us and mom. Gail instantly struck me as a woman with limitless energy – a keenly intelligent dynamo with an overabundant heart to match – an ideal representative for the nonprofit organization. After completing the paperwork and a brief interview, she informed us Jinx qualified for services. I couldn't believe it, we were actually going to have hands-on help!

Twice a week (Tuesdays and Thursdays), a home healthcare aide (instead of English servant Maggie!) would be coming to bathe mom, wash her hair and dress her. Afterward, a registered nurse would be arriving for an hour-long visit, to take her vitals, physically examine her, and answer any medical questions I had. Gail would be serving as our social worker, checking in with us every couple of weeks. A clergyman would also be at our disposal. Finally, real help was on its way! The kind I had asked mom's doctor about at the very beginning, when she had smugly replied, "Good luck with that."

Before leaving, Gail made sure I understood the terms of my mother's *conditional* acceptance by Hospice of the Valley. Jinx did not qualify for services based on her Alzheimer's, despite the disease being terminal. She had not reached "end stage," since she could still walk. Mom qualified due to the uncertain prognosis of her congestive heart failure. She would be "on probation" for 90 days. If in that time she didn't become end stage from one thing or the other, they would have to cut her loose. This was not HOV's preference; it was in accordance with their funding requirements.

That was fine with me – in 90 days we would have the ALTCS state subsidy approval for a nursing home. While I eagerly signed the hospice contract, Gail relayed another bit of exciting news to me: During the three months of service, we would be eligible for two, five-day respites while mom stayed at a memory-care facility, free of charge! Hallelujah! California, here we come!

The following Tuesday, my mom's bather arrived right on schedule. Sonia was a cheerful, fiftyish, Asian woman who, before coming inside, asked if I would help her bring in the supply box from her car.

"Supply box? What supply box?" I asked.

"We provide you with all the medical supplies you need," she informed me as we headed out to my driveway. Sonia moved with the speed and purpose of someone half her age. I could barely keep up with her and wondered why such a fit woman would need my help with a box. How big could it be?

It filled her entire trunk, that's how big! And it did indeed require both of us to carry the giant carton into the house. Sonia wasn't exaggerating about the supplies, either. The box contained packages of diapers, boxes of vinyl gloves, bottles of lotion, mouthwash, hand-sanitizer, perineal cleanser, soap, and tubes of diaper rash salve. We carried the incredibly generous care package into the house together.

I accompanied Sonia downstairs and introduced her to my mother. Mom gave her a quick, "Hello," and immediately returned to watching her TV show. I gave Sonia the grand tour of mom's bedroom and bathroom before leaving her on her own, to forge a relationship with the seemingly innocent little lady on the sofa.

"Give me a holler if you need help with anything. I'll be upstairs," I said.

Less than five minutes later, Sonia was shouting to me from below.

"I don't think Jinx wants to bathe today. She's refusing to get off the couch!"

I laughed out loud at my mother's lame attempt to control the situation. *Silly old lady.* I headed back downstairs to coach Sonia.

"Don't *ask* her," I said. "*Tell* her you're going to give her a bath. She doesn't have a choice. Make it sound fun and exciting…maybe try using a silly voice."

I summoned our British friend, Maggie, to demonstrate for Sonia.

"C'mon now young lady! It's time to go take a splash in the tubby! Get your lazy behind off the sofa this minute, or I'll get the fly-swatter, I will... Up you go, now!" I snatched mom's hand from her lap and pulled her to her feet.

Mom, the ever-devilish imp, stood there giggling, awaiting my next command.

Stepping aside, I handed off my naughty little kid to Sonia – so my mother could sense we were a team – and they proceeded to the bathroom without me. From that day forward, it was smooth sailing for our new aide – mom cooperated fully, and they became fast friends.

Sonia had a notable advantage; her lilting voice sounded similar to Lotus Flower's, my Asian, nail salon character whom mom adored. They both also called her "pretty lady" and "beautiful Jinx." And Sonia sure did make her look pretty! She French-braided mom's hair, adorned it with silk flowers, and wrapped her in her favorite, pink fleece jacket before leaving. What a warm, loving woman Sonia was. Our family treasured her.

Typically, within an hour after Sonia's visit, "Nurse Cindy" would arrive – always impeccably dressed – no medical scrubs and Crocs for her. Instead, she opted for breezy, flowing skirts (usually in shades of yellow), pressed white blouses, and strappy sandals. She was a shapely blonde, also fiftyish, who despite the sweltering Arizona heat, somehow always managed to look cool, composed, and professional.

Although friendly enough, Cindy maintained a serious, no-nonsense demeanor. Upon meeting my mother, she began rapidly dispensing medical advice to me.

"Her edema is very bad. You need to get her an ottoman as soon as possible, to elevate her feet while she's sitting. And you need to rub lotion on her swollen ankles throughout the day, to keep the skin supple. If that taut skin cracks open and fluid leaks out, the stench will be horrendous."

She didn't have to tell me twice! As soon as Cindy left, I headed over to Ross Dress for Less and found an ottoman for twelve bucks. I made sure mom's feet were up on that thing at all times, and I kept her ankles lubed! Cindy also recommended I purchase diabetic slippers (for swollen tootsies) and a personal blood-pressure machine for daily monitoring – which I promptly did. I couldn't help but wonder why none of my mother's doctors had suggested *any* of those things to me.

Cindy had thrown me a much-needed life preserver, with her medical expertise. She removed much of the nerve-wracking guesswork regarding mom's heart condition and new medications – which were now being delivered to my house, thanks to Hospice of the Valley.

Toward the end of June, Gail called to remind me about the extended respite included in our hospice service. She told me to pick a date, and she would arrange the whole thing for us. "As soon as possible!" I blurted out, over the phone.

The very next day, the ever-efficient Gail called back to say mom had a five-day, private room reservation secured at Wharton House, a memory care facility in Scottsdale. I made an immediate appointment to meet with the director, to make sure the place met with my approval.

The gorgeous, spacious, well-staffed home surpassed my highest expectations. I wish it had been in mom's price range, but the monthly cost (approximately $6,000 in 2013) was way beyond her means. They did not accept ALTCS state aid for payment.

What impressed me most about the place was how engaged the residents were in various staff-led activities. Some people were doing arts and crafts, some were playing board games, others were doing calisthenics, and a few folks were watching an Alfred Hitchcock movie in the living room.

Everybody was free to roam about the house as they would at home – the off-limits kitchen being the exception. Of course, nobody could go outside on their own either – special door codes prevented the residents from leaving the premises.

My biggest concern was the possibility my mother would be too afraid to stay with people she had never met before. How could I enjoy a relaxing get-away if she were scared or uncomfortable? I needed her to *want* to go there. While touring Wharton House, I ran a special request by the director, Mrs. Stovall. I had a plan for easing mom's potential fears, and I wondered if she and her staff would play along with my sneaky scheme. Mrs. Stovall loved the idea and said she'd be delighted to help me implement it. She also recommended I bring mom at the beginning of lunch, when all the residents would be gathered together in the dining room.

The day of our family respite had finally arrived, and it was time for me to put my plan into action: I sat down close to mom on the couch and flipped open my boating magazine, so she could see the colorful ocean pictures. Then I pointed to the photos and told her Harold, Caitlin, and I were going to go sailing in California for a few days.

"Do you like the ocean, Ma?" I knew the sea had always scared her.

"No," she shook her head. "I don't swim." Her face tightened.

"Oh, that's right. Would you rather go someplace else for a vacation?"

"Uh-huh," she nodded.

"I heard some very dear, old friends of yours miss you and want you to come visit them. Would you like to stay with your friends?"

"Oh yeah!" she smiled with noticeable relief now.

"Let's go pack for your trip then." I led her by the hand into her bedroom. Her small lavender suitcase was already open on the bed.

"Do you want to pick out some pretty outfits to wear on your vacation? Your friends can't wait to see you!"

Mom shuffled around the bedroom with excitement, grabbing random clothing pieces from her dresser drawers and closet – some of which made it into the suitcase, while others were discretely put back. (I felt it important she bring slacks and blouses that actually matched.)

Mrs. Stovall had also suggested we bring photos and personal items to make Jinx's room familiar and homey, so we packed a box full of those too: Two framed portraits of daddy, an embroidered lace pillow, and a few angel knickknacks. Mom was finally ready to head over to her "good friends' house."

As excited as I was for a relaxing getaway with my family, I couldn't seem to shake a bout of nerves on our drive to Wharton House. *What if mom was scared of her strange surroundings? What if she started crying?* When we arrived, I led mom along the walkway to the house – hoping Mrs. Stovall and her staff remembered my game plan.

Thankfully, I didn't have to wonder for very long. The front door suddenly burst open with a rush of "friends" hurrying out to greet my mother with smiles and outstretched arms. Each one took a turn hugging her (while I gave Mrs. Stovall a most grateful "thank you" hug).

"Jinx, our dear friend, welcome back!"

"How have you been? We've missed you!"

"Hello Jinx! We've been waiting for you!"

"Jinx, you haven't changed a bit!"

My mother embraced them all in the belief of being in the company of dear old friends. Undeniably, she was in the company of dear *new* friends.

"You're just in time for lunch, Jinx. Would you like to join everybody in the dining room?" Mrs. Stovall asked.

177

"Oh yeah!" Mom linked elbows with her escort and headed down the hallway with her entourage, while I happily followed behind. The parade was an incredible, celebratory exchange of greetings; mom waving to everyone she passed along the way and every single staff member shouting, "Hi Jinx! Welcome back!" I'd never been privy to such an amazing show of warmth and kindness by strangers. Their flawless performance, for the sole purpose of making an old woman feel at home, was more than my overjoyed heart could bear. I could relax now, assured the special people at Wharton house would take proper care of my mother.

While mom ate lunch with her "old" new friends, I unpacked her belongings in her room. I tried to arrange everything similar to the way it was at home – blouses hung in the closet, jammies and undies in the drawers, lotion on the bathroom sink, embroidered pillow on the bed, and angels on the dresser. Mrs. Stovall had instructed me to place something easily recognizable in the glass curio case located on the wall next to mom's door, to help her identify which room was hers during her stay. I knew a photo of "her Bill" would do the trick.

When I returned to the dining room, I found my celebrity mother had become the center of attention – the new girl everybody wanted to talk to. I joined her and her gang at their round table for some strawberry ice cream. All my qualms had dissolved. My new hero, Gail, had chosen the perfect place for mom. Before long, it was time for me to leave. I stood up and bent over to plant a kiss on mom's forehead.

"Okay, Ma. It looks like you're going to have a wonderful vacation here with your friends. I'll see you later, okay?"

Surrounded by her group of new pals she gleamed, "Oh yeah. Goodbye."

She waved me off with zero fanfare, bringing to mind Caitlin's first day of school, when, after entering the buzzing kindergarten classroom, she had

178

given her dad, grandmother, and me a similar brush-off. In both cases, all the unnecessary anxiety had belonged to me – not the loved one I was leaving.

During our family's San Diego sailing adventure, I didn't waste one second worrying about my mother's well-being. Nobody at Wharton House phoned me with any problems, and I had no urge to call them. Five days later, when I returned to retrieve mom, I greeted her with a giant bear hug and a necessary reminder of who I was.

"Hi Ma, it's me, your daughter Marlene. It's time to go home now."

"This *is* my home," she answered, flatly.

"We're going to your *other* house. You're a very rich lady – you have two houses."

"How 'bout that!" It was clearly news to her.

Mom's response was *exactly* what I'd hoped for; she didn't know her own home anymore. That would make my job so much easier in September when she would permanently become a resident of a skilled nursing facility – the exact one, yet to be determined.

My mother and I said our goodbyes to all the kind people at Wharton House and promised to return in a few weeks for our second respite. We made good on our promise, which turned out to be mom's final vacation with them.

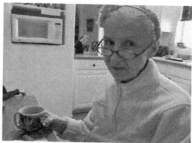

Jinx, all dolled up after Sonia's visit

A BITTERSWEET SUMMER

I knew the summer of 2013 would be my last one shared with mom; at home or anywhere. It had an ominous feel about it – her final countdown of months had begun. It reminded me of the first day of every summer vacation I had from school, as a kid. I needed to savor every second of it because September would arrive in the blink of an eye.

Arizona's hellfire summers are a whole different animal, though. The triple-digit temperatures are notoriously relentless. The poor fool without a pool (me!) is forced to spend most of June, July, and August (when overnight *lows* reach the 90's) inside their air-conditioned home, car, mall, or movie theater. Typically, I can't wait for summer to end, so I can go outside.

Such was not the case now. The oppressive heat still couldn't end soon enough for me, but September's imminent arrival held an emotional mixed bag regarding my mother's pending move to a nursing home. I wanted the mental peace and security that would come from relinquishing her care to fulltime medical professionals, but I dreaded her unavoidable departure from our home. Harold, Caitlin, and I had truly done all we could for her.

The help we received from Hospice of the Valley was a godsend. The mental and physical energy I derived from sharing my duties with Sonia and Cindy, directly translated into me spending more meaningful, quality time with mom. It didn't matter that most of it had to be spent indoors. Those three months became the most precious of all to me.

Mom and I enjoyed endless, leisurely hours together, igniting her lovely, long-ago memories. Reclined against a bank of pillows in her bed, we'd sit with one of her many old, black and white photo albums straddling our laps; mom slowly turning each delicate paper page, studying every snapshot like she was reliving it.

Curiously, mom could name all the people in each picture and in the next breath call me by one of her sister's names. I didn't mind if she saw me as Sophie, Margie, or Agnes, if it meant my family resemblance transported her back to a place and time she remembered, full of people she recognized and cherished.

Another stroll down memory lane we took almost daily, was perusing the scrapbook of Jinx's 80th surprise birthday party. It never failed to light up her face (and mine as well) every time we opened it together.

"Remember how surprised you were, Ma? Karen took you shopping all day, so we could get everything ready for the party. It was a BIG secret!"

"Oh yeah," she nodded, as her eyes moved from photo to photo.

"Our house was packed full of all the people who love you!"

"Uh-huh." Her smile widened as she studied the pictures intently. I wondered *exactly* what was going through her mind.

Weeks before the party, each invited guest had been asked to send a favorite memory of mom. Then Jaime compiled all their shared testimonials – the letters, poems, and photos – into a treasured keepsake album for the birthday girl. What a precious gift it turned out to be. At the time, we could never have imagined how invaluable it would become in the quest for evoking our mother's memories.

A few days after mom's birthday bash, I remember looking through the scrapbook with her and Billy. Sadly, I unknowingly forecasted her future.

"For your 90th birthday, we won't have to throw you a party, Ma," I joked. "We'll just show you *this* book and *tell* you we had a party because by then, you'll be too senile to know the difference!"

"Aint that the truth!" she laughed.

It was funny at the time.

Mom's eighth-grade graduation autograph book, from 1941, was another source for sparking memories. It must have held great significance to her, despite the many passing years; she kept the small purple booklet – embossed with a gold silhouette of a couple waltzing in the moonlight – instantly accessible, in the top drawer of her dresser. The pages were quite worn, but the corny poems inside (written by her classmates) were still clear enough for me to read to her:

- *When you are married and have a baby, don't let it join the navy.*
- *Yours 'til Italy becomes Hungary and fries Turkey in Greece.*
- *When you get married, and your husband gets cross, pick up the broom*
  and say, "I'm the boss!"
- *Yours 'til Jane Withers.*

And my all-time favorite:

Dear Sis,

> *No matter what they call you – Josie, Jinx, or anything else – you're still my sister, so what the heck!*

Your Big Sister,
Margie XXXX

I could read any poem and the first name of the friend who signed it – over seven decades ago – and amazingly, she'd tell me their last name:

Joe…Bartos

Dotty…Cherniak

Stiffy…Kozlowski

Bernice…Dykes

I could almost watch the gears turning in her head as she mentally traveled back to her grammar school days. The human brain is an incredible organ: My mother's memories from 70-years ago were locked tightly within her mind, while that morning's breakfast menu was already lost forever.

Mom also enjoyed visiting the cherished mementos found inside her jewelry boxes. Each time I'd place one on her lap, she'd open it with renewed curiosity – gasping at the treasures inside. Then she'd carefully pick out each one – a Virgin Mary medallion, a pocket watch, a keychain – and caress it with her fingertips before gently setting it down on the bedspread next to her. A heart-shaped locket, containing my dad's picture, elicited the same joyous response each time, "My boyfriend." I could see the deep love she still carried for him reflected in the faraway gaze of her moist eyes.

While hanging out at home with mom those three months, I thought I'd try reinstituting an old ritual we used to share, back when I was about nine-years-old, hoping maybe she'd remember it. Why not? I had nothing to lose.

While watching a favorite TV program, such as "The Carol Burnett Show" or "Rowan and Martin's Laugh-in," mom and I would divide the hour-long viewing time in the following way: I would brush her hair for the first 30 minutes, and she would tickle my bare back, with her long fingernails, for the remainder of the show.

I didn't know ANYBODY who shared that type of pleasant exchange with their mother, including any of my siblings. Ours was an exclusive arrangement. All I'd have to say to her was, "Scratch my back, Mommy?" and she'd reply, "Go get the hairbrush!"

183

Mom would plop herself down onto the living room floor, and I would sit behind her on the couch. Then she'd ooh and aah for a solid half-hour, while I slowly dragged the brush repeatedly through her thick, wavy hair. She especially liked when I reversed the strokes, running the brush up the back of her head. "Do that again," she'd say. "That gives me goosebumps!"

When it was my turn, I'd lie down next to her on the floor with my head in her lap. Then she'd slide her hand under the back of my pajama top and dance her nails around on my skin, eliciting similar goosebumps from me. Our session never lasted more than the duration of the TV show.

It seemed like a long shot, but I decided to try the same exchange while watching something of mom's choosing. This time, I suggested she sit on the edge of the sofa instead of the floor.

Mom selected the animated Disney classic, "Beauty and the Beast." Many moons ago, she and I had taken three-year-old Caitlin to see a "Disney on Ice" version of it, only to have our little stinker fart continuously on her grandmother's lap. Now it was just mom and me.

"Would you like me to brush your hair, Ma?"

"What for?" She looked confused.

"Because it feels really good. You'll like it."

"I guess so," she shrugged.

I sat behind her on the couch and ran the brush backward up through her hair, but it failed to produce any shivers or words of delight.

"Does that feel good?" I asked after a few minutes.

"I guess so." Her attention remained fixed on the cartoon playing in front of her. She didn't seem bothered by what I was doing, merely oblivious to it.

I ran the brush through her lifeless – but still thick – gray hair a few more times before setting it aside. Then, I stroked her back under her blouse with the tips of my fingers (my nails are too short!), certain I'd never get her to scratch mine.

"That tickles," she shivered and smiled over her shoulder at me.

I'll never know if anything I did triggered a memory for my mother or not. But it sure did spark wonderful ones for me.

Mom and I weren't total prisoners of our air-conditioned house that summer. We also took advantage of quite a few mild morning temps, scattering wild birdseed around the backyard to our favorite quail and mourning doves and blowing bubbles on the glider swing. Caitlin and I even managed to squeeze in a final trip to the Phoenix Zoo with her.

The three of us went in the very early morning hours, right after a cooling rain shower, rewarding us with increased animal activity. Our visit to the zoo the year before had been during its annual, winter holiday light event. Unfortunately, it is never great for viewing critters, since it takes place at night when they're all sleeping. Mom never noticed their absence; the musical colored-light displays and hot chocolate with marshmallows kept her happy.

Both trips had been equally fun, but what mainly sticks in my mind is how incredibly tough it was to push a grown woman in a wheelchair up and down the steep hills of our desert zoo. We made the most of it though; the three of us laughed our behinds off watching the crowds of frightened zoo patrons scatter in all directions as mom's downhill momentum increased beyond our control. "Watch out! We're coming through!" We were like three, rowdy kids on the loose!

Just like my childhood summers, the three months were over in the blink of an eye, and I couldn't have asked for a better one. That final, tender, bittersweet summer with my mother still stands as one of the most cherished seasons of my life.

THE FALL

The first day of autumn seemed a fitting one for mom's last day with us. Caitlin and I would be delivering her to Mountainside Nursing Center (in Phoenix) the following morning. I had a fun-filled day all planned for us, which included an ice cream outing once Harold and Caitlin returned home from their weekend camping trip.

It was early, about 7 o'clock. I went out to the driveway to retrieve the Sunday paper, while the pups gave the landscaping a morning sprinkle. I figured I'd let my mother sleep another hour or so, while I allowed myself a quiet, pensive breakfast. *Mom had only one more night to sleep in her own bed.* UGH! I had a feeling my whole day was going to be haunted by heavyhearted thoughts like that. As I headed downstairs to the kitchen, I casually glanced over the railing. And then I did a doubletake: Mom's lifeless form lay face-down, sprawled out on the floor below.

I stopped and stared, for a moment, in disbelief. It was real now; the horrible scene I had feared and imagined countless times. I had tried to do everything in my power to beat the odds of her falling. Only one more day and I would have. One. More. Day.

I felt strangely detached from the reality of it – almost like a spectator – as I watched myself float down the stairs in slow-motion. I didn't panic or hurry. I calmly stood over my mother and surveyed the situation. And THEN I freaked!

Oh my God! Is she alive? Is she breathing? How long has she been lying here? Did she trip? Did she break any bones? Can she move? Did she have a stroke or a heart attack? Check her pulse, you idiot!

I dropped to my knees beside my mother on the area rug – relieved she hadn't fallen *directly* onto the bare, flagstone floor – suddenly aware of my own erratic breathing. *Beat yourself up later, Marlene. Don't fall apart now!* I blinked my tears away and checked for mom's breath and pulse. She had both. Then slowly, she opened her eyes.

"Are you okay, Ma? Are you hurt? Can you move?" – way too many questions for her brain to process.

"I don't know." She stared blankly at me.

I called 911.

While waiting for emergency help to arrive, I remembered there are three questions you're supposed to ask a person who is possibly suffering a stroke. I thought, "What's your name?" might be one of them. Turns out it isn't, but that's all I could come up with.

"What's your name, Ma? Do you know your name?"

"Agnes," she replied. Agnes was her eldest sister.

I decided asking stroke questions would not help me determine whether or not mom's brain was getting oxygen. "Agnes" was not at all an abnormal answer for her to give me. Days later, when I researched the matter online, I discovered the three *correct* questions you're supposed to ask a possible stroke victim, none of which would have helped me in this instance:

1. Can you raise your arms and keep them up?
2. Can you smile?
3. Can you repeat a simple sentence?

I felt like I needed to do *something* before help arrived, but I didn't know what. I tried to roll mom onto her side, in an attempt to make her more comfortable, but I couldn't. Like a giant boulder, she wouldn't budge. Recalling nurse Fran's warning about "dead weight," I suddenly knew exactly what she meant. I decided against trying to move her, fearing a spinal injury or broken bones. Probably a good decision, since only five minutes later I had several Fountain Hills firemen by my side. I got out of the way and let them do their job. Mom was in capable hands now. Very sexy man hands, actually.

Despite the grave nature of the emergency situation, as I watched the rugged men tend to my mother, I couldn't help but notice the emergency team's striking good looks, like each one had stepped right out of the pages of a provocative, male calendar (The Burning Hot Hunks of Fountain Hills). My salacious fantasy triggered an immediate wave of guilt. *What kind of a perv am I?*

I looked on helplessly as they carefully lifted my mother onto a stretcher. Then I followed cautiously behind them as they carried her up the stairs. Standing in my driveway, while my heroes loaded her into their emergency vehicle, my body began to shake uncontrollably watching them drive off with her. I went back inside the house and wailed into my bed pillows.

At some point, I composed myself enough to contact everybody. Harold and Caitlin headed home from the mountains and my sibs headed to the emergency room.

On my drive to the hospital, I reflected on how useless medical alert devices are for people with dementia. Mom had worn one a year earlier, when the TV catch-phrase, "I've fallen, and I can't get up!" had prompted us to protect her with a home emergency system.

Jinx's electronic device hung from a lanyard around her neck, and initially gave our family a misleading sense of security. In the event of a fall, or any kind of emergency, all she'd have to do is press the large, red button. Easy peazy, right? Unfortunately, not true for anyone suffering with a cognitive disability. Mom couldn't comprehend its purpose and became intent on pressing the button for laughs. No amount of reasoning could stop the shenanigans, so I had to make the necklace "disappear." I couldn't allow her to continue signaling the company with false alarms.

To everyone's relief, the ER doctor informed us Jinx appeared to be okay. Remarkably, she had suffered no concussion, stroke, or broken bones. She would, however, need to be hospitalized for two or three days. When I phoned Mountainside Nursing Center to explain the delay in her admission to the administrator, he told me not to worry — he would take care of everything. He'd be in contact with the hospital and would arrange for mom to be transported directly to his facility upon her release.

He would take care of everything. How wonderfully comforting to hear somebody speak those words. I wasn't going to have to deliver mom to the nursing home after all; one less painful thing for me to worry about. But it soon dawned on me *exactly* what that meant: My mother would never return to our home again; she would never spend another night in her own bed; and we would never have our one last fun-filled day together. My heart sank.

When I got home, I went into mom's room and sat on the edge of her bed. As my eyes beheld the cozy surroundings, I realized the new transportation plan was actually a blessing. Now, my mother would be taken directly from a room in a hospital to a room in a nursing home, which were quite similar. The transition would be more seamless than the sharp contrast of going straight from her familiar, comfortable bedroom to the clinical environment of a nursing facility.

It would certainly be easier on Caitlin. No doubt she had been dreading the heart-breaking scenario of putting her grandma in the car, with her cute, purple suitcase and box full of assorted belongings, and driving her to the new place where she'd live out the final days of her life. I suspected my dear, brave daughter was doing it mostly for me; she knew I sure as hell couldn't bear to do it alone.

That evening, I suddenly remembered the conversation I'd had with Gail (from Hospice of the Valley), during her final home-visit, at the beginning of September. Only two weeks prior to my mother falling, HOV was forced to end their service to us. Gail informed me it wasn't the organization's choice to do so – Jinx simply hadn't met the required end-stage criteria. Neither her congestive heart failure nor her Alzheimer's symptoms had worsened *enough* during her 90-days probationary period. As Gail left my house that day, her parting statement to me proved prophetic:

"We hate to end services. Most of the time, within weeks after we leave, the patient ends up hospitalized."

OUR NEW LIVES

With Jinx's move-in date postponed to Thursday, Caitlin and I had three days to beautify mom's new room at Mountainside Nursing Center before her arrival. The minimal space – only half the size of her old bedroom – posed a bit of a decorating challenge. A floor-to-ceiling curtain divided the room into two; mom would be having a roommate and sharing the bathroom. Most of her belongings would not be following her to her new home.

Mountainside provided the basic furniture – bed, TV, dresser, and a couple of chairs. Caitlin and I struggled with the task of making mom's living space feel familiar and cozy despite the limited amount of personal belongings that could actually fit. Ultimately, we managed to spruce it up with many of the same items I had taken with us to Wharton House: Jinx's wedding portrait smiled at her from the nightstand, homemade art made by loved ones adorned the walls, and a scattering of angel knickknacks around the room watched over her. The addition of her embroidered pillows and stuffed animals made her new bed more comfy. Lastly, we stocked a dresser drawer with a few bags of spiced gumdrops and licorice.

Thursday morning, right on schedule, my mother arrived at the nursing home in a medical transport van. I greeted her at the entrance and enthusiastically wheeled her down the hallway to her new room. The limited exchange of words and blank expression provided no clue to her feelings.

Mom displayed no outward sign of confusion or fear as we traveled through the strange, new surroundings. She didn't acknowledge it as someplace she'd never been before. She made no mention of her room being different. Everything went smoothly – completely uneventful. The only difficult adjustment that first day turned out to be my own, when it came time for me to leave her there. I cried all the way home.

My tears were preferable to hers, however. The heartbreaking scenario of me leaving my little girl in a strange, scary place while she cried in confusion had thankfully been averted, due to a profound change in us both. I viewed her differently now, perhaps because I had relinquished her care to others. My little girl was gone. She was suddenly my terminally ill mother in a nursing home. As I resumed my original role of simply being Jinx's daughter, the transformation felt strangely natural, but it still hurt like hell.

My job was done. Officially, I was no longer my mother's caregiver. It took a while for me to reconcile such a foreign idea. Mom's overall welfare still occupied a large portion of my waking moments, except the daily, heavy burden of total responsibility had been lifted from my shoulders. But total relaxation still eluded me at home which, without mom in it, had a woeful emptiness about it.

We had *never* lived in our home without Jinx. We built the house and moved into it together, *with* her, when Caitlin was only three-years-old. The downstairs bedroom and bath were designed specifically for her. One-fourth of our family unit was suddenly MIA.

The entire bottom floor of the house cruelly reflected mom's absence. The fourth chair at the kitchen table – the one across from Caitlin – sat empty. Her TV in the family room remained dark and silent during the day; no more cartoons or Shirley Temple videos playing. Her side of the leather couch – the end cushion where she had planted herself every day – had a deep "butt dent" in it, like a heavy ghost still occupied the seat. We seriously wondered if it would ever spring back to normal. Not having mom around would clearly take some getting used to.

On the positive side, Harold, Caitlin, and I suddenly found ourselves with an abundance of free time on our hands, as our lives became our own once again. I was able to add more substitute teaching assignments to my week and complete the speech therapy program I had been chipping away at. Caitlin's employment and college schedule no longer depended on her grandmother's needs. Harold could return his full focus back to his construction business. The three of us immediately took another sailing vacation, this time without permission from anybody.

My mother's new life at Mountainside Nursing Center was an unqualified success, due *entirely* to the following two things: My strategic selection of the nursing facility and my steadfast belief in my brothers and sister.

Initially, the task of searching for the ideal, skilled nursing home for mom seemed pretty daunting to me; I didn't even know where to start. As it turned out, I was able to narrow down the field pretty quickly once I realized I only had three main criteria for the facility:

1. Acceptance of ALTCS co-payments. Mom could not afford the cost of *anyplace* on her meager monthly income alone.
2. A stellar reputation.
3. Close proximity to my siblings – a HUGE priority for me.

Mountainside Nursing Center fit the bill on all counts!

Without question, I knew planting mom in my siblings' "backyard" would be the best move for all concerned. The forty-mile, roundtrip drive to Fountain Hills had been prohibitive to them visiting mom. They needed their turn with her, to actively participate in her final months – to bring peace to *everyone* at the end.

Without them ever articulating it to me, I had suspected Karen, Billy, and Jaime needed and wanted the status quo reversed; their role expanded and mine diminished. My instinct turned out to be 100% correct, and then some. They ran with the ball! Between the three of them, mom had one or more visitors – day and night – during her entire stay at Mountainside. They floored me with their tireless, round-the-clock devotion.

Billy practically lived there. He would arrive early each morning and stay for most of the day. Oftentimes he'd leave and return again later. Jaime came almost every evening after work, with his wife and grown son. They'd visit during the dinner hour and took turns feeding mom when it became necessary. Karen lived close enough to walk over, which she did almost every day, sometimes several times a day, despite her own health issues. And they never came empty-handed – mom's room overflowed with toys, coloring books, flowers, cozy socks, and pretty blankets. Best of all, my siblings had the immense satisfaction of calling *me* to share the latest news of our mother – instead of the other way around.

Of course, I was never out of the loop anyway. As mom's power of attorney, the medical staff still reported all pertinent info directly to me, as did Sage Hospice, the organization that contracted with Mountainside Nursing Center to provide an extra layer of support for the seriously ill patients. Their team overlapped mom's nursing care with their own palliative care, at no extra charge to her.

No matter when I popped in to visit, I'd find one or more of my siblings already there. Sometimes I'd find Billy in the atrium, putting together preschool puzzles with mom; other times I'd encounter Jaime and his son, Michael, out front, touring the rose gardens with her; or I'd run into Karen and mom in the common room, petting the resident dogs or talking to the caged songbirds. The visits were always immensely better for me when they were there – the more company the better, since our mother had long ago lost her gift of gab.

Within her first week at Mountainside, Jinx acquired a new roommate. Caitlin and I met the feisty, little silver-haired woman named Opal, for the first time, while sitting with mom on the couch out in the common area. Opal was clearly not a happy camper. She had been a long-time resident of the assisted-living facility next-door, where her independent lifestyle had recently come to an end, due to a fall.

"I have to live over here with these sickos now, just because I fell down," she sneered.

"Oh, I'm sorry to hear that," I said. "This is my mom, Jinx. I guess you two will be roommates."

My mother greeted her with a friendly, "Hi!"

"Does she have dementia? So do I," Opal said matter-of-factly. "But mine isn't bad yet."

Then she pointed to an elderly woman slouched over in a wheelchair adjacent to us.

"Not as bad her. She eats paper! Why do I have to be in here with people like that? They're all nuts!"

The woman in the wheelchair didn't balk at Opal's accusation. She appeared completely oblivious, staring blankly at a potted plant.

That afternoon, Caitlin and I enjoyed a lively conversation with Opal. She seemed mentally "with it" and quite witty. She confessed to feeling lonely from not having enough visitors. We told her we would love to visit with her whenever we came to see Jinx.

"You can be my Aunt Opal! And I'll be your niece, Marlene. Would you like that?"

"I would love that! I'll be your Aunt Opal!" We both laughed and hugged each other.

The following week, when I visited mom, I peeked around the curtain dividing the room and waved at her.

"Hi, Aunt Opal! How ya doin' over there? Remember me, your niece, Marlene?"

"You're not my niece!" she snapped. "Stop lookin' at me. I'm tryin' to sleep!"

So much for Aunt Opal. Obviously, our previous meeting and conversation had escaped her memory, and for the remainder of my mother's stint as her roommate, she was barely civil toward any of us, except mom.

Opal resented the constant stream of visitors on mom's side of the room, prompting her to turn the TV volume way up to drown out the sound of our voices. That pissed-off Billy to no end. Besides verbally sparring with her, he actually resorted to hiding her TV remote when she left the room! This forced me to have to lecture him out in the hallway, on several occasions. But my words fell on deaf ears. No matter how many times I reminded him Opal suffered from the same mental illness as our mother, I got the same response.

"I don't care. She's still an old witch."

Jaime didn't like her either, but at least he didn't torment her. Karen and I felt sorry for her. Unlike our mother, Opal knew what was happening to her brain. She was clearly frustrated and angry at the world. She had once been an art teacher; a creative, talented educator. Her own lovely paintings decorated the walls on her side of the room. She still possessed most of her mental faculties, and she could still tend to her own needs. In Opal's mind, she didn't belong in a nursing home. I could only imagine what it must have been like for her, losing her privacy and strangers talking in her room all

196

day. Worst of all, knowing the woman on the other side of the curtain reflected her own cruel, imminent fate.

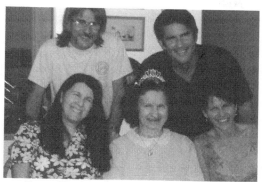

Jinx and her four kids at surprise 80th birthday party
Clockwise: *Billy, Jaime, me, mom, & Karen*

MOM'S HAPPY HOME

Contrary to most peoples' impressions of nursing homes, I didn't find the Mountainside Nursing Center depressing at all. The grim fact that it was the last leg of life's journey for many of its residents was certainly a downer to contemplate, but overall, it seemed an uplifting place to spend one's final days. Whenever I visited, I witnessed only inspirational professionals dedicated to providing compassionate care to seriously ill people – and always with a cheery smile. Jinx even had her own personal "Nurse Dreamy" – my nickname for the handsome young nursing student who bathed her.

There was always something entertaining going on at mom's new home. The center provided families with monthly calendars of scheduled activities, so they could participate as much as possible. My sibs and I were on board with that – enjoying all manner of arts and crafts classes, concerts, and dances along with our mother. MNC also welcomed a daily array of talented guests: Girls Scouts and school choirs sang for the residents; roaming magicians and jugglers traveled from room-to-room performing impressive tricks; serenading guitarists strolled the halls; pianists provided upbeat melodies in the dining room. Jinx had more on her social plate than ever before.

She also had greater access to her religious faith than she'd had in years. Every week, a Catholic priest would pop into her room and ask if she wanted to pray with him, which triggered deeply-ingrained words to spring forth from her memory:

"Hail Mary, full of grace. Our Lord is with thee..."

Sometimes, mom would recite the *entire* prayer. The human brain is truly astounding.

To my complete surprise, mom's doctor at Mountainside also informed us they'd be providing weekly physical, occupational, and speech therapy to her. It seemed odd to me, at first, since the entire staff knew she was now in the final stage of Alzheimer's. I skeptically questioned their intended game plan. What were they trying to do? Increase mom's vocabulary? Teach her how to brush her teeth? Fix her shuffling gait? Did the therapists really believe a person with the cognitive function of a two-year-old could re-learn those skills? It seemed like an obvious waste of time, money, and energy, since mom's total loss of all those abilities was already well underway.

Family members were encouraged to sit in on the therapy sessions, which we all did at various times. And I'm happy to admit, I couldn't have been more wrong about the amazing benefits. The unrealistic improvement of mom's skills was never the goal. The three therapists had a much higher motivation: Enhancing our mother's existence. What could be more important than that? They provided daily encouragement and validation necessary to nourish the human spirit. Their one-on-one lessons and interactions with Jinx gave her a much-needed sense of achievement and self-worth. Her completion of the simplest tasks — walking the length of a hallway or bouncing a ball — received glorious praise and high-fives. Mom basked in their attention. The therapists weren't trying to *teach* her anything — they were exercising and energizing her mind, body, and soul. They added purpose to her life. How does one even put a price on an invaluable service like that? It embarrassed me to think I had ever trivialized it or considered it otherwise.

I couldn't get over our good fortune in placing mom at Mountainside Nursing Center. It had exceeded my expectations for her care. Each month I sent them a paltry sum of $1,150 – mom's total income – minus $50 for personal expenses. ALTCS Medicaid subsidy covered the rest. Her Alzheimer's aside, Jinx Scribner was a lucky woman.

I didn't know it at the time, but I have since learned the state of Arizona has no requirements (as of this publication) for the caregivers of those with dementia. Many states have enacted legislation of licensing due to the complexity of care but not Arizona, where most its many senior citizens ironically prefer as little regulation (*aka public protection*) as possible. Here, facilities can hire staff and have them serving dementia patients the very next day, with zero training. As a precaution, I would recommend anybody interviewing potential caregivers request they be certified in Alzheimer's and dementia care.

Before we knew it, mom's first month at the MNC had flown by and Halloween was upon us. Our family was delighted to learn that neighborhood children were being invited to trick-or-treat at the nursing home, which was also hosting a Wizard of Oz themed party. Everybody was encouraged to wear costumes and dole out candy to the kiddies. That evening, we all attended the event with mom, and it was a total blast!

For at least two hours, a spirited parade of young Halloweeners snaked its way down the "yellow brick road," which ran through the common rooms of the home, collecting sweet treats from the residents and employees dressed as Oz characters. The hard-working, imaginative staff outdid themselves! Colorful, artistic backdrops had been painted on large drop-cloths which transformed each area into various scenes from the

200

movie; a Kansas farm with an approaching tornado, a sparkling Emerald City, the Scarecrow's cornfield, and a rainbow. Talk about elaborate – they went all out!

Mom rocked a Cleopatra-style wig, (made of shiny, magenta tinsel) along with her favorite, pink, mouse ears. I have to say she looked pretty bizarre! Our biggest challenge was convincing her to part with the candy she was supposed to hand out to the trick-or-treaters. Every time I looked over at her, she was stuffing another piece into her own mouth! At one point, instead of giving the treat to a child, mom actually reached into the kid's bag and snatched one out for herself! We more than compensated the confused youngster for our mother's transgression. That evening we all had a great time in "the merry old land of Oz!"

Despite all the fun going on around her, we hardly ever heard mom's laughter anymore. The latest evidence of her ongoing cognitive decline seemed most pronounced in her lack of vocal and facial expression. It's remarkable to think back on how precious the sound of that woman's laughter had become to us all. She showed little sign of emotion. That is, until her 34-year-old, granddaughter Stacy arrived from out-of-town.

Like all of Jinx's six grandkids, Stacy adored her grandma. She lived and worked in California as a theme park graphic designer but returned home regularly to see her parents (Karen and her husband Ken) and brother Shawn. This time, she spent part of each day at her grandmother's side, which prompted the most uproarious laughter I'd ever heard in the nursing home. Turned out, Stacy possessed something nobody else did – a fart noise app on her iPhone.

During most visits, we usually wheeled mom out to one of the cozy common rooms, next to the tiny songbirds. I'd often bring a photo album or mom's 80th birthday scrapbook from home, so we'd have something to reminisce over. Pictures from our Disneyland trip sometimes still got a snicker or two out of mom. But the real fun began as soon as Stacy pulled out her phone and opened the flatulence app.

The different fart categories were hilarious; trumpet fart, morning fart, diarrhea fart, squeak fart, and double fart. It didn't matter which one she picked, mom's faraway smile would instantly turn into the most wonderful, contagious, childlike laughter, and continue nonstop through the entire array of disgusting gassy sounds. Anybody within earshot of us must have thought we were one sick family – mentally, physically, or both.

NOVEMBER

Everything was humming along quite smoothly for Jinx — way better than I had ever imagined. With Arizona's punishing heat finally behind us, we all looked forward to taking mom out on some excursions in the glorious, 75-degree November weather. Just because her walking ability was on its last leg (pun intended), didn't mean we couldn't wheel her around the neighborhood for some sight-seeing and fresh air. Our family members were allowed to sign her out of Mountainside Nursing Center, for a few hours, almost anytime we wanted.

Besides its close proximity to my siblings, the location of MNC had another appealing advantage. It happened to be right around the corner from the last house my parents owned, where they had spent their final four years *together,* and where mom lived for another decade, before moving in with us. The facility was also down the street from the Desert Vista Mall and movie theater, places my mother had frequented hundreds of times. Through a lovely stroke of luck, Jinx's new home sat right in the middle of her old stomping grounds.

The DV Mall became the obvious choice for easy outings with mom, since it was only a 15-minute "roll" away. I usually recruited another family member to accompany me, in the event of an unforeseen problem arising. We always entered the mall through the food court, so mom could enjoy some non-nursing home lunch, first thing. She always chose either the McDonald's Happy Meal (gotta have that toy!) or a pizza slice.

203

After lunch, we'd take her through her favorite shops, lingering the longest in the candy store, and toy store. Of course, she'd always end up with a lollypop, or an ice cream cone along the way. Mom had very few words to express her joy by then, but her smiles and giggles were enough for us.

Whenever I visited my mother, she seemed in reasonably good spirits. Between the attentive staff, Sage Hospice, and my siblings, she was in many caring, competent hands. With the situation on autopilot, Caitlin and I made plans to get away for a weekend on the boat. But on the day before the trip, a nurse from MNC called with some bad news. "Jinx stood up to walk, fell, and most likely broke her other hip." She had no other details for me besides mom was in transit to the hospital.

I didn't blame anybody because I doubted anyone was negligent. Mom falling wasn't even a surprise to me. Afterall, she had the freedom to walk around the premises if she so chose. It was only a matter of time before she forgot how.

The first time Jinx broke her hip, in 2007, we wondered what she had tripped on in her bedroom to fall hard enough to break a bone. She said one moment she was standing, and the next moment she was face-down on the carpet. The doctor at the hospital immediately corrected our misconception: Mom's brittle pelvic bone had snapped, which in turn, resulted in her fall. I suspected this time, however, a disconnect within her brain rather than in her bone was the cause. The entire family gathered at the ER once again, only six weeks since her last hospitalization.

The attending physician confirmed my mother had indeed broken her other hip, and luckily, again, she had escaped further injury. He recommended surgery because she couldn't sit without excruciating pain. Over the years, I've been asked why we opted to have our terminally-ill mother's hip replaced. My answer is simple: Why would we want mom confined to a bed, flat on her back, during her remaining months? Her comfort and quality of life were still of paramount concern to all of us.

The doctor also informed us a family member needed to be present in the morning, to sign release forms and speak with the surgeon prior to the operation. To me, it was a no-brainer – Caitlin and I did not need to cancel our San Diego plans. I wasn't indispensable, so I reminded Karen she was second in command, according to mom's trust fund wishes. She could certainly sign papers and oversee the situation as well as I could, and I would unequivocally abide by all decisions she made on our mother's behalf.

Karen's initial apprehension prompted her husband Ken to quickly interject and assure me I could count on both of them to be there with mom, first thing in the morning. Jinx had been Ken's mother-in-law for 42 years by then, and he loved her like his own mother. His love and dedication to our family is why I regard him as nothing less than a true blood-brother.

At the time, I was not fully aware Karen was suffering from severe health problems of her own, brought on by the psychological strain of watching mom's mental deterioration. Much like our mother, my sister also always claims to be "good" or "fine" and prefers to keep her complaints to herself – never wishing to burden anyone. I knew she didn't feel 100% well, but since she hadn't elaborated any further, I assigned her to surgery duty. Being the reliable trooper that she is, she accepted without protest.

Caitlin and I headed for the coast the next day without worry. We were both on the same page about mom's surgery; we would not allow it to dampen our spirits or our good time. She and I had a realistic perspective regarding the woman we'd both spent years caring for together. Basically, our feelings on the matter were: *What could be the worst possible scenario? She*

doesn't come out of the anesthesia? Would that be so terrible? The countdown of her final
months had already begun.

Truthfully, the alternative – mom's Alzheimer's running its full course – frightened us way more than losing her during surgery. The uncertainty of her last days conjured up disturbing images of her lingering in a vegetative state. Plus, we both knew worrying to be a useless endeavor; she would go only when she was good and ready. Jinx Scribner had the constitution of a workhorse. The hip surgery she underwent, at age 80, had been a cakewalk for her, and we had a feeling she could easily do it again...with her eyes closed and backward.

Sure enough, around lunchtime, my purse started ringing. I pulled out my phone and saw the name *Soul Sistah* flashing on the screen – it was Karen, calling from the hospital.

"Mom's doing great! They already had her walking across the room!"

"Yep, that's our mother!" I laughed and relayed the news to Caitlin.

"Woohoo! Nothing keeps my grandma down!" she shouted, pumping her fist in the air. (I realize, now, nothing keeps my sister down either!)

We didn't need to talk about the obvious: Despite her new hip, mom's walking days were surely over. No doubt, the nursing home staff would insist she use a wheelchair from here on in. The risk and liability of her falling again would be far too great, since she lacked the full mental capacity to reliably do so. If they didn't automatically resign my mother's fanny to a wheelchair, I would demand it.

A week or so after Jinx's surgery, all of her therapies – speech, occupational, and physical – were halted due to the loss of her receptive language. Mom could no longer comprehend the directions given to her by the therapists, rendering her incapable of doing the exercises and activities. Again, not a surprise to me. We had been expecting it because she was

206

becoming less and less responsive to all stimuli. On the bright side, it opened her daily schedule for extra outings.

One afternoon, when I had mom out for a neighborhood spin, I thought maybe seeing her old house again might spark some memories, so I wheeled her over to the sidewalk in front of the last home she had shared with her husband.

I set the brake on the chair, intent on a leisurely visit; one which would give mom an unrushed opportunity to really study the place. The single-story, block house had held special meaning to her. It was my parents' first and only brand new home. They had watched every phase of its construction, and they were immensely proud of it. I was hoping it would stir an emotional reaction the way her photo albums and jewelry box trinkets had. Actually, *any* hint of recognition from her would have made me rejoice.

"Here's our old house, Ma! Remember when we lived there?"

"No."

She stared at it. No emotion. No sign of recollection.

"Look how big your two carob trees are now!"

Nothing.

I pointed to her kitchen window.

"Remember cooking in that kitchen, Ma?"

"No." The same flat voice.

"Well, I do. You made delicious meals!"

I pointed to her stone garden wall.

"Remember all the pretty flowers you planted in the flowerbed?"

"Uh-uh," she shook her head.

"All the snapdragons and roses? Yours were the most beautiful on the whole street!"

Vacant stare.

Over the course of twenty years, mom and I had stopped at the house dozens of times together, usually for only a couple minutes, the visit pretty much the same each time. We'd sit in the car and remark on the two most notable changes: How the trim was so much prettier painted red, "when we owned it," and how the side of the house looked bare without "daddy's roadrunner" on it.

Daddy's roadrunner decorated almost half the west-facing exterior wall. Incredibly, my father had pruned the Pyracantha vine into the improbable shape of a giant roadrunner; not just any old roadrunner, but *the* roadrunner from the Wile E. Coyote and Roadrunner cartoons. Springtime covered the "bird" in white flowers and summer dressed it in a suit of bright orange berries. Passing motorists actually stopped to take pictures of it! Back then, reminiscing with my mother in front of our old house inevitably ended in warm hearts and smiles as we pulled away from the curb.

This time, she and I lingered in front of the house for at least 20 minutes, while I kept plugging away, attempting to evoke the past. "Remember daddy's roadrunner bush?" But it was no use. Nothing prompted the slightest flicker of recognition; not a word; not a smile. My heart ached with defeat. Even so, I did not consider my unsuccessful attempts a waste of time. Just because mom couldn't display the emotions I desperately longed for didn't mean the feelings weren't somewhere deep within her mind and heart.

I remained crouched on the sidewalk beside her, holding her hand, overcome by my own vivid memories of my parents' once-blissful life at that address – holding back a flood of tears I would surely release later at home. It was time to move on now. Rising to my feet, I kissed her on the cheek before continuing on our journey around the familiar (to me, anyway) streets of the neighborhood known as – believe it or not – Roadrunner Estates.

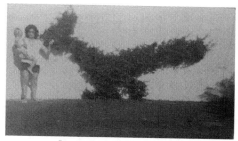

Jinx and "daddy's roadrunner"

The month of November ended with a wonderful, but poignant, celebration – our final Thanksgiving dinner with mom. We all knew it was the last one. It had to be, since she was in the final stage of Alzheimer's now. Nobody needed to say it. Instead, we all focused on the simple joy of having her with us for a lovely afternoon at Karen and Ken's house.

Mom seemed to enjoy being the special guest of honor. She had eleven devoted servants buzzing around her throughout the momentous meal. The heaping plates full of food placed in front of her would have satisfied King Henry VIII. We brought her everything short of a bejeweled goblet of wine!

The conversation at the table soon turned to our memorable Disneyland trip and the Thanksgiving dinner we enjoyed at the Rainforest Café, only two years ago.

"That sure was fun, huh Mom?" Jaime put his arm around her.

"Yeah," mom replied, without expression.

We all felt so grateful we took her when we did.

HAPPY HOLIDAYS?

The holiday season brought a festive air to the nursing home, with glittering ornaments, caroling school groups, and cookie parties in the dining area. Our family made sure Jinx's room was well-decorated for Christmas, complete with a small, tabletop tree in the corner – decked out in twinkling colored lights and the requisite angel on top.

During December, we all made extra trips to the DV mall with mom, including one for her 87th birthday. That little lady could still put away an impressive amount of pizza and root beer! A joyous, unspoken gratitude permeated the day; Jinx was still with us. Yahoo!

We spent as much time as possible at the mall that month because the vibrant sights and sounds of the holiday stimulated mom like nothing else, seeming to spur her back to life. We could actually see intermittent flashes of wonder in Jinx's eyes, especially as she caught sight of the 30-foot-tall Christmas tree, sparkling in gold garland. And Andy Williams' singing *It's the Most Wonderful Time of the Year* (in almost every store), stirred a bit of rhythmic head bobbing. We even witnessed a return of some humor.

On one of our most memorable mall outings, my siblings and I wheeled mom past Santa's workshop, the big man himself waved at Jinx and called out in his jolliest voice, "Ho Ho Ho! Have you been good this year, young lady?"

Mom smiled and replied, "Nope."

Karen interjected, "Don't you believe her!"

Then he asked her, "Is there something special you want me to bring you for Christmas?"

She chuckled a little, "No."

Then I pointed at mom, "Watch out for this one, Santa. She's a big jokester."

"Yep." Mom's smile widened into her familiar, mischievous smart-ass grin, and we all had a belly laugh with our naughty little elf. It was great having her back – even temporarily.

As December 25th drew near, our family excitedly made plans for celebrating the holiday with mom. But two days before Christmas, I received *another* call from one of mom's nurses. Jinx had been rushed to the emergency room, *again*. This time, I was told, it had something to do with a severe salt imbalance. *What did that mean?* The details were vague. For a third time, in as many months, our family headed to the hospital.

While Harold searched for a parking spot with Caitlin, I dashed into the ER entrance. A busy orderly directed me to mom's room at the end of a long corridor, but as soon as I set foot in the doorway, I could see he was clearly mistaken. The disfigured, shriveled woman in the bed bore no resemblance to mom. I abruptly did an about-face and went to look for somebody who could give me the correct room number.

As I was leaving, Jaime and Billy somberly approached me with ashen faces, visibly shaken.

"Did you see mom?" Jaime's tone was grave.

"No, I'm still trying to find her. Do you know where she is?"

"Yeah, she's in there," Billy said. They both looked pointedly at the room I'd just come out of.

"That's what the guy said, but have you been in there? That's not mom."

"Yeah, we've been in there," Jaime was adamant. "It's her alright. She's wearing the ring that has our birthstones in it."

Billy nodded in agreement. They both blinked away tears.

I darted back inside the room and inspected the woman in the bed more closely. She looked exactly like every picture I'd ever seen of an unwrapped mummy. *This person cannot possibly be our mother!* I frantically examined her right hand. The guys *had* to be wrong. But there it was…on the stranger's finger; the filigree band inset with our birthstones – an aquamarine, diamond, amethyst, and ruby.

There was no mistaking that ring. Karen bought it for mom when my brothers and I were still kids. The stones weren't real, but the sentimental value sure was. I had removed my mother's wedding rings and other jewelry – for safe keeping – the day she moved into the nursing home, but the band of birthstones wouldn't budge over her bony knuckle.

I couldn't speak. Standing there in shock, I was horrified beyond words. My mind couldn't comprehend the hideousness of what my eyes beheld. It was straight out of a "Ripley's Believe It or Not!" museum. The woman's severely wrinkled flesh and bizarre protruding buck teeth, were in sharp contrast to our mother's smooth skin and snug-fitting dentures. Jinx was altogether unrecognizable.

By the time I turned around, Harold and Caitlin were entering the room, followed by Karen, Ken, Shawn and Stacy. The whole group instantly became distraught at the sight of mom.

"Jesus Christ, what the hell happened to Ma?" Ken cried out.

"That's grandma? Oh my God!" All the grandkids were sobbing.

As if on cue, a doctor arrived to provide us with some much-needed answers. He assured us Josephine Scribner would pull through, but she was barely conscious, and suffering from something called *hypernatremia dehydration* – a deficit of total body water relative to total body salt. In other

212

words, the concentration of sodium in her blood was way too high, and the amount of water in her body was dangerously low.

He recited a list of factors which could have led to mom's condition: The diuretics being administered for her edema (caused by the congestive heart failure), her severe dementia, and failing kidneys. He also explained her jutting teeth; mom's gums had shrunk from the extreme dehydration! Although Jinx's condition was terribly serious, the doctor expected a full recovery.

All any of us could do in the moment was stand by helplessly and watch the intravenous fluids flow into mom's arm, in the hope of seeing her withered body replenished back to normal.

"Will she be out for Christmas?" Karen sniffled into her ball of tissues.

"I'm awaiting some test results." The doctor did not sound optimistic.

As he started to leave the room, I informed him my mother wore dentures and asked if he could please remove them from her mouth, which he promptly did. *Why hadn't somebody already done so for her?* Mom looked dreadful enough as it was – she didn't need giant rodent teeth too!

All day long, the doctor's words played on a continuous loop in my brain. He had given us a list of possible reasons for mom's horrendous condition, but no insight into *exactly how* the salt imbalance might have occurred. I wondered if it was the result of a proverbial "perfect storm" – a critical number of negative factors, simultaneously causing a disastrous event. None of us were satisfied with his incomplete explanation. It occurred to me that perhaps he was purposely trying to avoid unfairly implicating the nursing home.

It was impossible for us not to conclude mom's caretakers at the home dropped the ball somewhere along the line. Jinx couldn't request a drink or necessarily even recognize her own thirst. The responsibility fell to her nurses to make sure she was properly hydrated, which obviously they had not. I planned to Google *hypernatremia dehydration* as soon as I got home.

Our family remained at mom's side in the ER for several grim hours, awaiting her transfer to a hospital room. While I was preoccupied with signing a mountain of medical paperwork to sign, my brother-in-law, Ken, noticed Caitlin emotionally breaking down. The sight of her dear grandmother, appearing to be in the throes of rigor mortis, was too much for her to bear. I heard Ken whisper to her, "Hey Cait, you wanna take a walk down to the cafeteria with me?" He hugged her gently to his chest, and she crumpled into him – her tears coming harder now – as he lovingly escorted her from the room. I'll never forget his kindness and sensitivity, on that dreadful day, and I know Caitlin won't either.

Finally in her own room, Jinx's skin elasticity returned along with her natural appearance. She was semiconscious, but in a seriously weakened state from the severe shock to her system. Word soon came down from the doctor – mom would not be coming home for Christmas.

Karen took the news the worst of anyone, with giant sobs into her husband's shoulder. Christmas is *the* most important day of the year to her; she lives for it. She sets money aside for the holiday all year long and spends literally the first 24 days of December doing nothing but decorating, shopping, and wrapping presents. My sister is a true embodiment of the Christmas spirit. Nothing could kill the magic of the holiday she held so dear. Except something like this – her mother, lying deathly ill in a hospital bed. It was a particularly, extra gut-wrenching blow to Karen.

We all hugged each other and headed to our respective homes with the heaviest of hearts, resigned to our fate of Christmas Day without Jinx.

That evening, I began my online research into mom's condition and discovered a wealth of information on the subject of *hypernatremia dehydration* on several websites, including Healthline and the Mayo Clinic's. I was surprised to learn the general geriatric population is predisposed to developing the complication, as a result of common physiological changes due to aging; specifically, their decrease in thirst sensitivity and body water content.

In younger people, water accounts for 60-65% of body weight. For senior citizens it drops to about 50%, and even lower for women. Aging kidneys also present a problem, since their chief role is to maintain the proper balance of water and sodium in the body. As the kidneys lose their ability to concentrate the urine, the capacity to retain water also decreases. Dementia patients are at an even greater risk due to their impaired thirst mechanism.

Compound all of the above with residing in a nursing home – where anybody can easily be overlooked – and you have a recipe for disaster.

The more I read, the angrier I got – at everybody and everything – including mom, who had harbored a lifelong aversion to drinking water. I could never convince her of its importance to her overall health. She always gave me the same lame, ignorant excuse:

"My coffee has water in it. That's enough for me."

No matter how many times I told her coffee was a stimulant and a diuretic which caused her to lose extra fluid by peeing more frequently, she still refused to drink water simply because she didn't like it. In the handful of years I took care of my mother, overseeing her hydration *personally*, she probably drank more water and sports drinks than in all her other years combined. And wouldn't you know it, as soon as I relinquished the responsibility to someone else, mom winds up in the hospital looking like a strip of beef jerky.

215

My research also revealed *hypernatremia* is oftentimes a condition of neglect, for which a nursing facility can be held legally responsible. But litigation was not something I wanted to pursue. To me, not every human error justifies a lawsuit. Had the error resulted in mom's death, however, I'm sure I would have thought differently about the need for further investigation and accountability.

As much as I wanted to assign specific blame to somebody, too many unknowns muddled Jinx's case. Even though she obviously had not been hydrated sufficiently, there was no way of knowing exactly what transpired. Were her nurses negligent in providing enough water? *Or* did they bring her an ample amount, but didn't stay to watch her drink it all? *Or* was mom's daily water requirement underestimated due to her aging kidneys malfunctioning?

It was mind-boggling to contemplate all the possibilities. I wondered exactly how one goes about monitoring a dementia patient's water intake, 24/7? Maybe Jinx poured some of her water into a plant or flower vase? She no longer received one-on-one personal attention, like she did at home. She had three shifts of different people essentially "tag-teaming" her care; critical information being passed from one worker to the next, under the unrealistic assumption it's intercepted and interpreted properly *every* time.

In any relay race, it's certainly not uncommon for the baton to be dropped while being handed to the next runner. Do I think somebody "dropped a baton" at MNC regarding my mother's fluid intake? Yes, I do. But mom also had at least a dozen other strikes against her as well, preventing me from concluding *pointed* neglect. Ultimately, for my own peace of mind, I decided to pin the blame on "a perfect storm."

Our family did not cancel any of our Christmas traditions that year; we simply rearranged everything to revolve around our cherished matriarch.

216

We brought her tiny decorated tree from the nursing home to the hospital to make her room as festive as possible. On Christmas Eve night, we all gathered around her bed with the presents we bought her, trying to act cheerful – which was not an easy task, given mom's frail appearance. Alarmingly, she now had a *nasogastric* feeding tube plugged into her nose, secured to her precious face with tape.

The thin, transparent tube looked similar to many oxygen breathing devices I'd seen. A nurse told us Jinx was having trouble swallowing, and it was the preferred method for delivering nutrition rather than an IV, since it went directly to the digestive tract instead of into the blood vessels. Our family assumed her need for a feeding tube was temporary. Nobody told us otherwise, and none of us thought to ask if mom's inability to swallow was a permanent condition. We were all mainly focused on trying to bring her some Christmas joy. I don't remember my mother speaking at all that evening, but I vaguely recall a few weak smiles from her. I suspect my brain might have purposely blocked out much of the sorrowful visit.

I was also suffering from a painful, raging, sinus infection, and most likely a fever, so I wore a surgical mask and kept a respectable distance away from my sick mother. A part of me was grateful for the protective face covering – it hid my tear-soaked cheeks and spared me from having to sustain the strained phony smile everyone else had plastered on their face. I wished I still had some Lexipro. The "happy pills" had worked wonders three Christmases ago.

Before leaving the hospital, I gave mom a parting kiss on the feet – through furry Christmas socks – instead of her face (again, to guard her health). When I said, "Goodnight Ma," I felt certain it was for the very last time. My overwhelming sense of despair and loss caused me to totally break down bawling before I could reach the elevator.

The following day, Christmas dinner at Karen and Ken's, brought us all together again. Jinx's absence from the family's holiday gathering hung heavily in the air. Nobody had their usual appetite – worry and tension can be very filling. Thankfully, there had been no word from the hospital. For us, no news was good news. We planned an early meal, so we could all visit mom afterward, before it got late.

Jarringly, in the middle of dinner, my phone rang. The solemn faces surrounding me said it all – we knew it had to be the hospital. Every person who would call me on Christmas Day was sitting right there at the table. The phone rang again. I desperately didn't want to answer the damn thing. Quickly pushing back my chair, I dashed into the next room to take the call.

I don't know why I did that. It seems silly now, since the meal was already disrupted. The phone conversation – the one my family surely strained to overhear – was going to be shared with them anyway. Everyone was palpably on edge. Perhaps, in running from the room, I felt I could somehow run from the news, as well.

THE FEEDING TUBE DECISION

Do we have to decide this right now? Over Christmas dinner?" I asked.

Another blow. A doctor from the hospital called to inform me of the dire need to install a *permanent* feeding tube into my mother's stomach as soon as possible.

"Mrs. Scribner chokes on her food when swallowing and aspirates when drinking. Inhaling liquids into her lungs puts her at serious risk for pneumonia," she explained. "We would like to do the surgery first thing tomorrow morning."

"My mother is going to have to eat *all* her food through a feeding tube in her stomach, for the remainder of her days? I need to talk this over with my family. We're eating dinner, right now, so I'll have to call you back."

I returned to the table and stared at my plate for a minute, trying to gather my thoughts. I needed to accurately and coherently convey the information to everybody and get their opinions. Personally, I didn't know what my *own* opinion was yet. Everyone had overheard enough of my phone conversation to know mom had another serious problem. They wasted no time in grilling me.

"What's going on with mom now?"

"Is grandma okay?"

"What did the doctor say?"

I relayed the distressing message to them, as calmly as I could, to keep from upsetting anybody more than necessary. The doctor had bombarded me with the news of mom's latest grave condition yet left me with so many unanswered questions. I didn't have many facts or any insight to give them which, to me, meant thorough research needed to be done on the subject in order to make an educated decision. But the doctor insisted the situation was urgent.

"So...what do you think? What should we do?" I asked everyone.

My family sat in stunned silence, searching for answers in each other's eyes.

Harold and Caitlin were the first ones to weigh in with their position. They felt the feeding tube procedure was a bad idea; one which would only postpone the inevitable. Plus, it was certainly not something to decide under pressure. Everyone agreed with them, but picturing Jinx choking or drowning on her food was horrible to contemplate. Jaime, Karen, and Billy voted in favor of the surgery. I was on the fence, leaning more against the tube but also afraid *not* to do it.

"Mom won't ever be able to savor the taste of food in her mouth anymore," was my principle argument. "I wouldn't want to live like that. But is it worth dying of pneumonia?"

We could hardly imagine a more depressing holiday dinner conversation. The passionate debate continued around the table. I'm proud to say my family remained logical and reasonable during the emotional discussion, and it never became heated. We all wanted what was best for Jinx — we just didn't know what that was.

Be it good or bad, the sanctity of Christmas carried an enormous amount of weight regarding our decision. We all knew mom's time on earth was seriously limited, but her dying on or around December 25th, in such a gruesome way, was a tragedy we all hoped to avoid. Daddy's unexpected passing already indelibly marked Thanksgiving. And although my nephew Shawn was too selfless to mention it, his birthday was in three days.

Technically, as her POA, I had the final say, though I certainly did not relish it nor even want it. In the end, I reasoned it this way: Three out of four of mom's children had strong opinions in favor of the feeding tube. Since her fourth child, me, remained undecided, I felt it only fair to defer to them. Apprehensively, I called the doctor back and gave consent for the surgery, known as a *gastrostomy*.

After dinner, we all returned to the hospital, to mom's bedside.

"Merry Christmas!" We all shouted as the eleven of us filed into her tiny room.

Mom looked every bit as frail as she had 24 hours prior. Except now, she sported huge pillow-like mittens on both hands – resembling cartoonish Mickey Mouse gloves – to prevent her from grabbing and yanking the nasogastric tube from her nose, which we were told she had done twice that day. Poor mom. My heart ached for her. The damn thing had to be miserably uncomfortable, and of course, impossible for her to comprehend.

During our visit, we learned from one of the nurses that a nasogastric tube is *always* only a temporary solution, therefore, the doctors must have concluded mom's inability to swallow properly was a permanent condition, warranting the gastrostomy. We had hoped to learn more about the procedure by speaking personally with a doctor that evening, but being Christmas, staffing was scarce and there were none to be found. I went over to the nurses' station and sincerely thanked them all for spending their holiday with my mother instead of their own loved ones.

I remember very little about the visit, except it felt as equally bleak and sorrowful as the night before: More disingenuous smiles, a sad little twinkling tree on the table, my mother propped up in bed with a tube threaded through her nose, my sinus infection raging under the surgical mask, and more tears. I had sentenced my mother to an invasive surgical procedure, and I had no clue if it was really in her best interest or even truly necessary. My thoughts kept returning to the idea of mom *never* tasting food in her mouth again. I couldn't make peace with it. My head was about to explode from both the physical (sinus) and mental pressure.

The following morning, a doctor phoned to say the gastrostomy went fine, and mom was doing well. She would be returning to the nursing home within a couple days. Positive news, for sure, but nothing about the call lifted my spirits. I'm not sure they were "liftable."

The most appalling phone call from the hospital, however, came the next afternoon. It was a completely different doctor, one with whom I had never previously spoken. And her blatant tone of disgust was unlike *any* I had ever heard in a medical professional.

"Why would you subject your sick mother to a surgical feeding tube procedure when she is at the end of her life? Don't you understand? All Mrs. Scribner should be getting now is palliative care. Your only concern should be making her as comfortable as possible. You need to stop doing things to prolong her life, just to make yourself feel better."

I couldn't believe my ears. She continued to scold me until I cut her off midsentence.

"Enough!" I blurted out, barely able to restrain my rage. "Excuse me? Trying to *prolong* her life? That's the last thing my family wants to do. We only okayed the procedure because a doctor, at *your* hospital, strongly advised us to do it to prevent her imminent, excruciating, choking death. Are you saying the doctor steered us wrong? Did your hospital perform an unnecessary surgery on my mother? My family and I were urged to make this decision over Christmas dinner, no less."

Before I could get her name, the rude woman quickly hung up, offering me no explanation, nor apology. Her unprofessional, emotional demeanor gave me pause to wonder if she was really a doctor. Regretfully, I was remiss in keeping track of the many physicians and surgeons who treated mom at the hospital. I should have kept a log of names.

By the weekend, Jinx was transported back to Mountainside Nursing Center. Shortly after mom's return, Dr. Merritt (mom's doctor at the nursing home), phoned me. Her voice was gentle and compassionate, but her inquiry about mom's surgery revealed the same dismay and underlying message as the disparaging hospital doctor who had called.

"I'm curious as to why you opted for this procedure when your mother is at end-stage Alzheimer's?"

The doctor's polite tone and demeanor compelled me to contain my anger and respond with patience. I calmly recounted the whole story for her, while she listened attentively and without interruption. She didn't blame me, but she expressed frustration and regret over the hospital directing and pressuring us the way it had. Deep down I was seething, but I couldn't take it out on her. She was only the messenger.

Dr. Merritt stated that for end-of-life patients, whose bodies are shutting down, a feeding tube is usually not the best way to go. When I asked her about the danger of mom choking or inhaling food (as it had been described to me), she said the preferred solution was to puree all her solid foods and thicken all liquids, allowing mom to comfortably eat and drink with no feeding tube necessary. Translation – the surgery had been unnecessary. The doctor's next remark made me see red:

"Eventually, her feeding tube will more than likely get clogged and have to be removed. It's difficult for some medications, like pills, to pass through it."

"What?! Why would a doctor advise such a procedure, especially with such urgency?"

She had no answer for me, but rather, seemed embarrassed by certain members of her profession. She apologized profusely for the unfortunate situation.

While my stomach churned from the doctor's revelations, my mind raced with suspicion. From the very beginning of Jinx's illness, I had held more than a few reservations about the physicians I had encountered, especially regarding what I perceived as unnecessary testing. In my opinion, mom's comprehensive medical coverage invited abuse, and now that she had both Medicare *and* Medicaid (the state subsidy) – double coverage – it felt like "open season." The feeding tube debacle cemented my already-cynical beliefs about the broken healthcare system and the ethics of some doctors and hospitals.

All we could do was move forward. We had to live with our choice, so our family made the best of it. Mom's meals were being fed to her via the tube each day, but we all agreed she could still safely eat certain things orally such as gelato and Otter Pops. Since Dr. Merritt had mentioned pureed foods as an acceptable option, we assumed anything with the consistency of ice cream would be harmless. Karen brought some type of frozen treat for mom every day and provided close supervision as she ate it. Mom's eyes lit up with every bite and no coughing or choking occurred. I could mentally tolerate the harshness of the feeding tube for my mother as long as she could still enjoy the pleasure of tasting food in her mouth.

Incredibly, three weeks after its installation, mom's feeding tube became clogged from her medicine and promptly removed – exactly as the doctor predicted. Not exactly a happy start to the New Year. While researching feeding tubes online (after it was too late for Jinx), I unearthed the following information from sites such as AgingCare and DailyCaring:

224

- In older adults with advanced dementia, the evidence does not support the use of feeding tubes.
- The use of a tube can cause discomfort and may fail to dampen feelings of hunger or thirst.
- Feeding tubes can interfere with a peaceful and natural death.
- At the end of life, the body is shutting down and is often unable to process the food being fed via the tube. This results in food backing up into the lungs or the membrane lining the abdominal cavity. In the case of the latter, peritonitis – a life-threatening infection – usually occurs. It also means feeding tubes don't provide 100 percent protection against aspiration pneumonia.
- Feeding tubes can shift out of place, also causing peritonitis.

Please understand, I don't have the medical expertise to advise for or against a feeding tube for anybody's loved one. Each case must be evaluated individually. The only advice I'm qualified to give you is to research the subject *before* the need arises, so an unemotional, informed decision can be made. I wish I had done so. The potential risks and possible trauma to my mother had conveniently been omitted from the doctor's urgent recommendation on Christmas Day.

Soon after mom's feeding tube became blocked, the nursing home gave us *more* bad news: Jinx had peritonitis in the membrane lining of her abdomen.

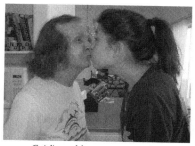

Caitlin and her granny smooching

225

TWILIGHT TIME

It was hard to ignore mom's swollen, extended belly – a third trimester pregnancy looks weird on an 87-year-old woman. She displayed no outward signs of pain, but we knew she couldn't possibly be comfortable. During a visit with our mother, Dr. Merritt appeared in the doorway and asked Karen and me to join her in the atrium garden for a chat. The doctor got straight to the point and did not sugar-coat her words.

"Jinx's condition is life-threatening. She will probably not survive the peritonitis. If I were you, I would not make any imminent travel plans. You should advise the rest of your family to stay close to home and prepare yourselves for the end."

My sister and I remained outside, mulling over the doctor's warning while trying to regain our composure. The truth about the feeding tube was obvious now; it had been a colossal and tragic mistake. The doctors in the hospital had surely known mom was *actively dying* – a medical term for someone in the final phase of life. But instead of providing compassionate palliative care, they heartlessly recommended a harmful, gratuitous surgery. It seems money never fails to motivate certain individuals and institutions.

Intravenous antibiotics were now being administered to Jinx for the peritonitis. All we could do now was hope for a quick, relatively painless passing. Under the dire circumstances, my niece Stacy postponed her trip home to California.

Three tense weeks passed, with the entire family braced for the worst, but by the end of January, it was clear mom wasn't going anywhere. The peritonitis went away, we all returned to our "normal" routines, and Stacy flew back to Los Angeles. I told you mom had the constitution of a workhorse!

Mom survived the infection but had totally lost the ability to feed herself by then. On a positive note, she was eating her meals orally again, in the manner Dr. Merritt had originally described. To avoid aspiration, a thickening agent was added to all her liquids and to prevent choking, her solid foods were being pureed. Not everything needed altering; she could eat mashed potatoes and gravy with ease. The solution was astoundingly simple and, again, underscored the hideously unnecessary feeding tube procedure.

Jinx was now being served her meals in a much smaller, more private dining area. Usually, there were about 8-10 other residents in there along with her, who required the same level of assistance. My siblings did not like the idea of their mother having to wait for her nourishment (God bless 'em!), so they diligently fed her *every* meal themselves and personally inspected all her liquids to ensure the proper thickness. As an added precaution, we also kept a canister of powdered *Thick-It* (available at all drug stores) on hand in her room, to make our own necessary adjustments if necessary.

Feeding mom was a slow and arduous process, each time requiring an entire hour in the narrow dining room. Despite the cramped quarters, at any given time Jinx had at least two family members sharing the duty. Sometimes there were five or six of us at her table at once, requiring extra chairs being brought in. My family usually turned the whole affair into an impromptu party, filling the room with laughter, even though mom's had ceased – even for zany fart noises. But every once in a while, she still gifted us with her endearing little smile.

Incredibly, my mother still maintained her deep-seated disdain for eating fish. Pureed fish might look different, but it still smells and tastes like fish. Mom would push it away every time – sticking out a pouty lip in protest. Naturally, her hawkish children immediately sent it back to the kitchen in exchange for something else to her liking.

Our family seemed to have one unified mission now: Mom had provided her kids (and grandkids too) with nourishment when we were little, and it was our turn to reciprocate. Of course, as children, *we* didn't have the option of not eating stuff we didn't want. We didn't dare send food "back to the kitchen," and pouty lip refusals got *us* nowhere. All we could do was inconspicuously slip the offensive food – for me, usually peas – to our dog. I'm pretty sure mom pretended not to notice, allowing us to believe we were getting away with something.

The circle of life was unfolding before my eyes. Watching Caitlin feed her grandmother sent my memory wheels spinning back to Thanksgiving Day, 1990, when Jinx flew to San Diego to spend the holiday with us. Her newest grandchild, Caitlin, was turning 5-months-old. We didn't own a camcorder yet – they cost about $1,000 back then – so we rented one for twenty-four hours. The VHS tape we recorded on that special day is so valuable to me, I keep it locked in our home safe.

The end product is an absolutely riveting video (perfect for insomniacs) of our darling new daughter, Caitlin Rose: Caitlin sleeping, Caitlin swinging, Caitlin being diapered, Caitlin rolling on the floor, Caitlin sucking her toes, Caitlin in the bathtub. There is also plenty of footage of the proud new parents, the doting grandma, our cocker spaniel, and pet rabbit. Out of all of it, my favorite segment is of my mother feeding Caitlin jarred baby food.

It wasn't just any old routine feeding; it was Caitlin's first introduction to solid food, specifically Gerber's applesauce. Mom asked if she could be the one to give it to her, and I happily allowed her the pleasure of doing so, while I played cameraman.

The scene takes place in the living room of our small house. Mom is sitting on the floor with Caitlin (strapped in her baby carrier) in front of her. Harold is on the couch dividing his attention between watching the feeding of his daughter and an old episode of *Bonanza* on TV.

The next ten minutes of footage is zoomed in on mom dishing out the golden goo, on a tiny spoon, into the awaiting "baby bird's" gaping mouth. Caitlin kicks her tiny feet with excitement. Mom makes kissing noises and says, "Dat a girl!" and "Hey, stop kicking me, you!" Applesauce runs down the baby's chin, grandma catches it in the spoon, and shovels it back in. When the jar is empty, Jinx gently wipes her new granddaughter's face and gives her a loud smooch. An indelible bond has been forged between them. Priceless.

My happy memories still came with piercing moments of heartache.

By February, Jinx was tiring easily, spending more time in her room. During visits, we all grew weary of the TV always being on and longed for some other type of entertainment for us. I had read how beneficial listening to familiar music was to dementia patients, so I asked Caitlin if she would help her techno-dork mother create a CD of her grandmother's favorite songs. The two of us brainstormed the playlist and put together an eclectic mix: Mom and daddy's love songs — *Lara's Theme (Somewhere My Love)*, *Spanish Eyes*, *Hawaiian Wedding Song*, and *Twilight Time*, as well as some upbeat, fun tunes — Shirley Temple singing *Animal Cracker's in My Soup* and a lively polka, *Who Stole the Kishka?* Caitlin and her grandma used to polka around the kitchen to that one.

We kept a copy of the CD in Jinx's room along with her boombox, so anybody visiting could play it for her. Mom obviously enjoyed it, noticeably perking up whenever she heard the familiar songs. Disgruntled roommate, Opal, was not a fan, however. Inevitably, we'd hear her moan, "Oh, not again!" from the other side of the curtain divider, and within a few minutes she'd shuffle out of the room in a snit.

Although we could still occasionally observe a tiny spark of our mother's personality, we knew she was really only existing at that point. Jinx couldn't walk, talk, toilet, swallow properly, wash, dress, or feed herself. She couldn't even stand on her own. She had to be lifted – by a burly male nurse – in and out of her bed. Mom reminded me of a life-size doll as various people moved her around in the same way I had once done with my Barbies.

By April, Jinx was spending most of each day lying on her back in bed. Pillows were needed to prop her into a sitting position, otherwise she flopped over. In her wheelchair, she took on the appearance of a limp ragdoll, slouched over to one side, barely able to hold her head up. Mom was eating noticeably less food, causing her muscles to weaken.

Easter and Stacy's 35th birthday fell on the third Sunday of April, so she returned to Arizona, once again, for what normally would have been a celebratory weekend. The family lunched at a restaurant near the nursing home, before gathering for a solemn, subdued, Easter visit with mom. We brought cards and balloons with us and plenty of stiff upper-lipped smiles, but she was barely with us that day.

In the dining room, Jinx's head drooped forward, her eyes sunken and yellow. She couldn't eat any of her holiday dinner. She coughed and choked on each spoonful, a grim sign her ability to swallow was completely gone. We wheeled her back to her room and called for someone to come and lift her into bed. Mom's CD of favorite songs lulled her instantly asleep. Each member of the family took a few minutes alone with her to say goodbye in private, fearing it was our last visit with mom.

Jinx did not pass away on that Easter Sunday. More days passed. *What the hell was she waiting for?* An IV drip provided all nourishment now, since she could no longer take food orally. Completely confined to her bed, she also had a steady stream of oxygen flowing into her nose. My mother's medical directive stated no *extraordinary* measures should be taken to prolong her life, such as a ventilator or any type of machine. It also included a Do Not Resuscitate (DNR) order. Were the IV and oxygen extraordinary measures? The answers to such questions no longer seemed black and white. It was torturous to see mom like that. How does one reconcile such a contradiction of feelings – the simultaneous desire and dread of a loved one's death?

I watched the nurses diligently buzzing around my mother; changing her diaper, checking her vitals, cleaning her with a washcloth – like a newborn in a nursery. I wondered if her soul, trapped inside her earthly body, was struggling to leave.

The Friday following Easter, I got a call from the Sage Hospice clergywoman, Ellen. We had never met but we had spoken a few times by phone. She had visited with mom many times during the past seven months and knew she was nearing the end. Ellen called to ask me if I had any requests for her – of a religious nature – such as a special prayer. The poor unsuspecting woman, compassionately reaching out to me, never saw it coming; something within me suddenly snapped, and I let loose an angry rant of biblical proportions. Not directed at Ellen, personally – more like at the *whole* world.

"My mother is practically a vegetable now! An animal in her condition would be humanely put to sleep. How is this acceptable? I guess there's still

231

too much money to be made off her! Mom would have wanted her life ended the moment Harold, Caitlin and I started intimate care of her. Nothing would have been more humiliating to that proud, modest woman. I can't bear it another minute – seeing her lifeless…but still alive."

Ellen listened patiently, without interrupting. I carried on, almost hysterically, for several minutes about how people should have the right to die with dignity; a right most certainly denied my mother. At the end of my tirade, Ellen said she understood exactly what I wanted her to pray for and promised to do so. I found that curious, since I didn't have the slightest clue myself. I apologized for my rude outburst and told her I'd deeply appreciate her exercising any connections she had with "the powers that be."

The next morning, Saturday, Dr. Merritt called to tell me Jinx went into a coma during the night; she would pass soon. I cried tears of gratitude. *Thank you, dear Ellen.*

Mom's room could have used a revolving door that day as friends and family came to pay their last respects. Billy's daughters, Sherri and Candi, drove down from Northern Arizona with their children, filling Jinx's room to the brim. Even her niece, Marie, flew in from Colorado for a final chat with her dear aunt.

"Everyone is waiting for you in heaven, Aunt Josie – your mom, pop, brother, sisters, and handsome husband. It's time for you to join them now."

That afternoon, a Catholic priest administered last rites to my mother.

It was an extremely long, draining day…and yet it wasn't nearly long enough. Mom appeared to be sleeping peacefully, with no IV or oxygen now. I slipped the CD of favorite songs into the boombox one last time for her. Everyone gathered at her bedside, smiling bravely through their tears; each song sparking cherished memories of the beloved woman we were about to lose. We each privately said our final farewells to her, once again. This time, we all made sure to emphasize it was okay for her to go because her work here was done.

Alone with mom now, the Platter's *Twilight Time* played quietly in the background, as I sat beside her on the bed, holding her aged, but beautiful, hands in mine; the hard-working, healing hands of a selfless wife and mother.

Heavenly shades of night are falling, it's twilight time.

I leaned in closer and caressed her hair and forehead with my fingers, remembering how the once soft, brown waves framed her gentle face.

Out of the mist your voice is calling, it's twilight time.

Then I laid my head on her chest to listen – one last time – for the faint sound of mom's loving heart. I swallowed hard, and took a couple slow, deep, breaths before speaking softly into her ear. My tears spilled freely as I thanked my mother for all her tender love and care, for modeling a perfect marriage, and for shaping the strong woman I had become.

When purple-colored curtains mark the end of day

Finally, I pressed my lips tightly onto hers, lingering as long as I could before saying, "I love you, Mom. Daddy is waiting for you now – go give your Bill a kiss."

I'll hear you tonight at twilight time.

The next morning, Sunday, April 27th, I awoke to the sound of my phone at 5:30. Instantly shooting upright in bed, I snatched the device from the nightstand and let it ring again in the palm of my hand, pausing to steel myself. I had mentally prepared for the moment hundreds of times: The many mornings I approached her bedroom door; whenever she dozed too soundly on the couch; each time I left her hospital bedside; every kiss

233

goodbye at the nursing home. For God's sake, I had even begged for it –
Please relieve my mother already! But I guess we're never really prepared, are we?

Relief had finally come. To mom and to all of us. It was time now. Time
to let her go.

Goodnight, Ma.

All My Love,

Marlene

EPILOGUE

I like to lightheartedly describe June 14, 2014 as the day my father "came out of the closet." His cremated remains – which had been stored on the top shelf of mom's bedroom closet since 1982 – would finally be combined with his beloved wife's and dispersed into the natural beauty of Arizona's landscape.

Six weeks after mom's passing, our family gathered for a small, informal ceremony on what would have been the 67th wedding anniversary of Jinx and Bill. My parents had never specified exactly where they wanted their final resting place to be. My mother's request was simple – "Just put us someplace pretty." Nobody had a preference, except Jaime, who suggested a favorite fishing spot of his, in a picturesque area known as Arizona Rim Country. Everyone agreed the location sounded like the perfect final resting place.

It was an idyllic site indeed; in the cool shade of a pine forest, with the scenic Verde River winding through it. Dramatic, vermilion cliff walls provided a majestic, cathedral-like effect for a glorious celebration of our parents' lives. We planned an informal picnic lunch of Kentucky Fried Chicken – Jinx and Bill's favorite fast food.

Our group of fourteen included my siblings, our spouses, our children, a teenage grandson of Billy's, and me. The CD we made for mom provided the music for our feast and memorial service on the spectacular riverbank.

Our family spent the afternoon enjoying the peacefulness of the woods as we shared our heartfelt and humorous memories of mom and daddy.

Before the commencement of the ceremony, I couldn't help but notice the stark difference between my parents' cremains: Daddy's reminded me of a 5 lb. sack of flour and contained rock-size chunks of bone fragments; Mom's looked more like a one pound bag of coffee, with contents resembling finely ground seashells.

I wondered if the difference was due to a change in the cremation process over the last three decades or the fact mom had significantly less bone mass at the end than daddy. He had left a hardy, 58-year-old body behind; she, a ravaged 87-year-old frame riddled with osteoporosis.

At last, the time had come for us all to bid farewell to them. We gathered solemnly around the grandest, most stately pine in the forest, and after digging a small hole at the base, Jaime slowly poured their ashes in. Next, he tenderly and tearfully stirred them together with the tip of the spade and covered them with soft soil. A large stone was then placed on top; one painted with their names, *Jinx & Bill,* inside of a heart.

While my parents' favorite love song, *Somewhere My Love,* rang out from the hillside, our family made our way down to the water's edge with a smaller portion of their ashes. Standing on the riverbank, with the magnificent cliff walls towering over us, we blended the beloved couple with the water, allowing them to become part of the gentle, summer flow of the Verde River.

Someday, we'll meet again, my love

At the end of that emotional June day, the extended Scribner clan somberly headed out of the woods. Bill and Jinx were finally together again, but it felt strangely unsettling to us, leaving their remains, all alone, out in the wilderness – as if they were still alive. But as we all hugged each other goodbye, through tears and smiles, the realization of what *actually* remained of Bill and Jinx came into razor-sharp focus for me: We were the living embodiment – three generations – of my parents' durable, familial bond of love and commitment. We weren't leaving them behind at all; we would forever be joined together *through* them.

* * * * * * * * *

Caring for Jinx brought out the very best in all of us. To be sure, it brought me closer than ever to my treasured siblings – Karen, Billy, and Jaime. We see each other through different eyes now; we have each borne witness to each other's strength, dedication, and devotion. Since our mother's passing, we say, "I love you" to each other with more ease and frequency. What an incredibly lovely testament to her.

In the end, did I ever get to know the private woman, Josephine Ann Scribner? Not exactly; not in the way I had long hoped for. The intimate relationship I had spent years seeking – the one where mom shared her innermost secrets with me – existed only in my imagination. Somewhere along the way, during my time as her caregiver, it lost its importance to me as a new relationship emerged from a more mature perspective; one which grew from understanding, compassion, gratitude, and forgiveness. The mother-daughter relationship, I once considered superficial, had been replaced by a deeper, more meaningful bond. As intimate as any two people could share.

237

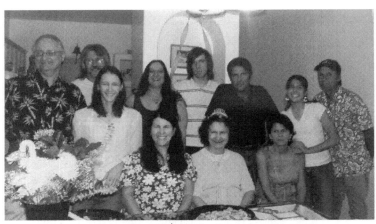

Jinx's 80th Birthday Party – December 2006
Starting Top Left: *Ken, Billy, Stacy, Sundie, Michael, Jaime, Caitlin, Harold, Karen, Mom, & Me. Shawn took the photo*

RESOURCES AT YOUR FINGERTIPS
(For All Types of Dementia)

- Alzheimer's Association
  (800) 272-3900 – 24-hour Caregiver Hotline
  Alz.org

- Alzheimer's Foundation of America
  (866) 232-8484 – National Toll-free Hotline
  Alzfdn.org

- National Hospice and palliative Care Organization (NHPCO)
  (703) 837-1500
  Nhpco.org

- American Association of Retired Persons (AARP)
  Aarp.org/health/dementia

- Mayo Clinic
  Mayoclinic.org/diseases-conditions/dementia

- American Speech-Language-Hearing Association (ASHA)
  Asha.org

- Born to Talk an Introduction to Speech and Language Development
  by Merle R. Howard and Lloyd M. Hulit

- HealthLine
  Healthline.com

- Team Select Home Care
  Teamselecthh.com

- Medline Plus: Trusted Health Information for You
  MedlinePlus.gov

- WebMD
  WebMd.com

FOR ARIZONA RESIDENTS

- <u>Hospice of the Valley</u>
  (602) 892-9630
  Hov.org

- <u>Arizona Long Term Care System (ALTCS)</u>
  Health Insurance for Individuals Who Require Nursing Home Level of Care
  (888) 621-6880
  Azahcccs.gov

ABOUT THE AUTHOR

Marlene Jaxon
Author – Speaker – Advocate

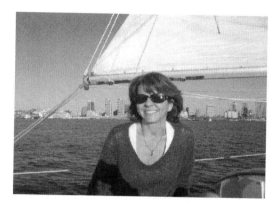

Marlene resides with her husband in Arizona, in a house they designed and built together 26 years ago – along with their melodious miniature schnauzer, Roxanne. She is the proud mother of a treasured daughter and wonderful, new son-in-law. Although there are many aspects of Arizona to appreciate, the New Jersey native will always have ocean water in her soul and prefers to spend as much time as possible by the sea, in her adopted home state of California. Besides writing, her interests include sailing, world travel, hiking, archery, playing piano and guitar.

www.MarleneJaxon.com

Made in the USA
San Bernardino, CA
17 January 2020